**Antenatal
Disorders
for the
MRCOG
and Beyond**

Published titles in the MRCOG and Beyond series

Neonatology for the MRCOG *by Peter Dear and Simon Newell*

Menstrual Problems for the MRCOG *by Mary Ann Lumsden, Jane Norman and Hilary Critchley*

Gynaecological and Obstetric Pathology for the MRCOG *by Harold Fox and C. Hilary Buckley, with a chapter on Cervical Cytology by Dulcie V. Coleman*

Management of Infertility for the MRCOG and Beyond *by Allan A. Templeton et al.*

Forthcoming titles in the series

Early Pregnancy Issues

Fetal Medicine

Gynaecological Oncology

Gynaecological Urology

Intrapartum Care

Molecular Medicine

Paediatric and Adolescent Gynaecology

Reproductive Endocrinology

Antenatal Disorders for the MRCOG and Beyond

Andrew J. Thomson
MB, ChB, MD, MRCOG

Honorary Senior Lecturer in Obstetrics and Gynaecology, Glasgow University, and Consultant in Obstetrics and Gynaecology, Royal Alexandra Hospital, Corsebar Road, Paisley PA2 9PN, UK

Ian A. Greer
MB, ChB, MD, FRCP(Glas), FRCP(Ed), FRCOG, MFFP

Regius Professor and Head of Department of Obstetrics and Gynaecology, Glasgow University, Department of Obstetrics and Gynaecology, Glasgow Royal Infirmary, 10 Alexandra Parade, Queen Elizabeth Building, Glasgow, G31 2ER, UK

Series Editor: Peter Milton

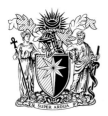

RCOG Press

First published 2000.
Reprinted 2004

ISBN 1–900364–36-0

Published by the **RCOG Press** at the
Royal College of Obstetricians and Gynaecologists
27 Sussex Place, Regent's Park
London NW1 4RG

Registered charity No. 213280

Cover illustration: Colour flow Doppler ultrasound showing two umbilical arteries and a single umbilical vein in a normal umbilical cord
RCOG Editor: Jane Moody

Typesetting: Saxon Graphics Limited, Derby, UK
Printing: Cromwell Press Ltd, Aintree Avenue, White Horse Business Park, Trowbridge, Wiltshire BA14 0XB

Acknowledgements

The authors are grateful to Dr Alan Mathers and Dr Fiona McKenzie, both of Glasgow Royal Maternity Hospital, for providing many of the figures

Contents

Preface

John Ballantyne of Edinburgh demonstrated the value of antenatal care in the early 1900s, prior to which time there was virtually no provision made for this very important area of obstetric practice. In his publication *Antenatal pathology and hygiene: the embryo and the fetus*, which was published in 1904, he predicted many of today's prenatal and perinatal developments. Antenatal care was subsequently established in the UK but was still, of course, only rarely available throughout much of the world. The pattern of antenatal care in the UK changed little from Ballantyne's pioneering days until the last few years of the 20th century. During this time we have seen important developments in the delivery of routine antenatal care, which has now devolved largely to the community, and more precise means of fetal assessment. These techniques are thoroughly reviewed in the early chapters of this extremely useful volume. In subsequent chapters complications of pregnancy and medical disorders are deal with succinctly and thoroughly. Although the contribution made by physicians to the care of pregnant women with medical disorders is of the greatest importance, such patients are generally cared for by physicians and obstetricians working together. The contribution made by midwives and general practitioners to antenatal care has rightly increased over the years and this volume will prove extremely valuable to anyone striving to provide the best possible care for pregnant women.

Peter Milton
September 2000

1 Antenatal care and risk assessment

Introduction

Patterns and provision of antenatal care have changed enormously in recent years in response to the opinions of consumers, providers, professional associations and government reports. During pregnancy, most women remain well and require little formal medical input. For them, pregnancy is a physiological process. However, some women develop complications with significant morbidity or mortality for their baby and, occasionally, for themselves. Providers of antenatal care must be able to distinguish between these two groups of women and arrange with them an appropriate and personalised plan of care.

Epidemiological and observational studies have demonstrated that women who receive antenatal care have better pregnancy outcomes with lower maternal and perinatal mortality. These studies have also demonstrated an association between the number of antenatal visits and pregnancy outcomes after controlling for confounding factors, such as the length of gestation. However, recent work has been directed to the quality of antenatal visits rather than the quantity. It has been suggested that more effective care could be provided by fewer goal-orientated visits, particularly focused on the elements of antenatal care which have been scientifically proven to be effective and have an impact on outcomes.

Who should provide antenatal care?

In recent years, the issue of who should provide antenatal care has been widely debated. A study carried out in Scotland in 1989 (Tucker et al. 1996) showed that obstetricians, general practitioners and midwives working together (shared care) provided 97% of antenatal care. Lately, midwife-managed programmes or antenatal care by providers other than a consultant obstetrician (usually general practitioners and midwives working together) have been implemented for women considered at low risk of pregnancy complications. These models of care have been compared with consultant-led shared care in randomised controlled trials.

> **AIMS OF ANTENATAL CARE**
> - To provide advice, reassurance, education and support for the woman and her family.
> - To deal with the minor ailments of pregnancy, such as abdominal discomfort, heartburn, backache, haemorrhoids, nausea and vomiting and varicose veins.
> - To screen for, diagnose and manage pre-existing maternal disorders, such as diabetes, heart disease and infection. This screening programme should continue through pregnancy to confirm that the woman remains well throughout pregnancy.
> - To identify women at risk of maternal or fetal complications during pregnancy and, where possible, to prevent these from adversely affecting the health of the mother or her baby.
> - To promptly identify and treat any new medical or obstetric problems arising in pregnancy.
> - To plan for labour and delivery, care of the newborn and future general and reproductive health.

These trials show that midwife-managed care, as opposed to consultant-led shared care, had similar, or in some cases, more favourable outcomes. A randomised controlled trial comparing midwife-managed care with shared care at the Glasgow Royal Maternity Hospital (Turnbull *et al.* 1996) found that women in the midwife-managed group were less likely to have induction of labour and less likely to have an episiotomy. In other studies, care by general practitioners and midwives resulted in:

- individual women seeing fewer carers
- fewer non-attendances and hospital admissions
- marginally fewer routine hospital visits than with consultant-led shared care.

Furthermore, lower salary costs and enhanced women's satisfaction were obtained by providing midwives' clinics.

The involvement of the consultant obstetrician in the antenatal care of low-risk women has been challenged. Some obstetricians advocate that consultants should manage only those women with complicated pregnancies. It has been argued that:

- most women with uncomplicated pregnancies do not want to see an obstetrician
- general practitioners and midwives are able to fulfil most of the aims of antenatal care

- studies have demonstrated that the outcome of pregnancies in low-risk women is no better when obstetricians are involved.

Further, it has been proposed that the specialty should develop so that all obstetricians should have expertise in ultrasound evaluation of the fetus, manage common medical disorders complicating pregnancy and have skills in high-dependency obstetric management. In contrast, others have argued that women with complicated pregnancies must be managed by someone who is regularly exposed to normal and abnormal patterns of pregnancy and labour. Normal pregnancy is a retrospective diagnosis and many women initially categorised as 'low risk' will develop complications during their pregnancy. Tucker *et al.* (1996) found that over half of 'low-risk' women developed some complication during their pregnancy and had to be seen by an obstetrician. As many of these complications are minor, reversible or require only a small amount of medical input, such women may be returned to low-risk care after obstetric assessment and treatment. While some obstetricians might argue that it would be more appropriate and less stressful for these women if the obstetrician whom they have already met continued their care, in practical terms this is difficult to deliver owing to the volume of patients. Interestingly, a survey of obstetricians working alongside a midwife-managed maternity unit showed that the majority of obstetricians acknowledged the need for change and expressed positive attitudes to midwifery care (Cheyne *et al.* 1995).

In 1995, the Scottish Office published a report by the Clinical Resource and Audit Group/Scottish Health Management Efficiency Group (CRAG/SCOTMEG) Working Group on Maternity Services, summarised in Table 1.1. This report included an integrated model of antenatal care, which aimed firstly to improve continuity and prevent duplication by reducing the number of antenatal visits, and, secondly, to improve quality by integrating antenatal education and clinical care in a single visit. The model stresses the need for integration of care, with each professional fulfilling his or her role. There were similar conclusions drawn in the *Changing Childbirth* report (Department of Health 1993).

The number of antenatal visits

In the 1920s, when a national system of antenatal clinics with a uniform pattern of visits and procedures was introduced, the average number of antenatal visits during each pregnancy was 14. Studies in Aberdeen have critically evaluated the number of antenatal visits undertaken by women and have shown that a reduction from 11.2 visits in 1975 to 8.7 in 1981–82 was not associated with any adverse effects in clinical outcome.

Table 1.1 Summary of the CRAG/SCOTMEG Working Group report on antenatal care programmes

- Each woman should have a maternity care co-ordinator

- Each woman should have a choice of maternity care co-ordinator

- The maternity care co-ordinator is responsible for planning care and ensuring that follow-up action is taken

- Antenatal care should be personal to each woman and care should be tailored to meet the individual woman's needs

- Quality should be improved by integrating antenatal education and clinical care in a single visit

- Continuity should be improved and duplication prevented by reducing the number of carers and the number of antenatal visits

- Participation and co-operation should be encouraged between all those involved in the care programme: the woman, midwife, general practitioner and obstetrician

- Integrated care should allow each professional to appropriately fulfil their roles

Despite recommendations made by the Royal College of Obstetricians and Gynaecologists in 1982 that there should be fewer antenatal visits, the Chief Scientist's Office in Scotland (Howie *et al.* 1991) reported that the average number of antenatal visits was 15, that visits were not tailored to individual's needs and that women considered to be at low risk were being seen as frequently as women considered to be in the 'high risk' category. More recently, randomised controlled trials have demonstrated that, in developed countries with well-established maternity services, small reductions in the number of antenatal visits (two visits less) are compatible with good perinatal outcomes. One trial conducted in a developing country (Harare, Zimbabwe), in which a significant reduction in the number of visits was achieved (six visits in the standard care group and four visits in the intervention group), appears to support this conclusion, at least in that particular setting (Munjanja *et al.* 1996).

In London, Sikorski and colleagues (1996) found that women having more antenatal visits had more ultrasound scans and more antenatal day admissions, although this increased use of resources was not associated with any other measurable clinical effect, beneficial or otherwise. However, more women randomised to the reduced schedule of antenatal visits were dissatisfied with the number of visits and over half of the women in this group felt that some of the gaps between antenatal visits were too long. The authors conclude that more flexible approaches to the provision of psychosocial support and the reassurance of women about fetal well-being may be needed if reduced schedules of antenatal visits are to be introduced. Furthermore, the particular problem of pre-eclampsia can develop suddenly and progress rapidly. If there is to be a reduced frequency of antenatal visits, then not only is appropriate risk assessment required but also women need to be educated with regard to the importance of antenatal care in general and the development of specific symptoms and signs in particular.

Contents of the antenatal visit

Current programmes of antenatal care have evolved from models developed in the first half of the 20th century. Although antenatal care has been modified to incorporate advances in medical knowledge and new technology, these developments have been introduced without proper scientific evaluation. The contents of antenatal care visits are more ritualistic, rather than based on clinical evidence. The contents of the booking visit are shown in Table 1.2. To take full advantage of antenatal care, women should book in the first trimester or early second trimester. It is well recognised that 'late bookers' are at increased risk of adverse pregnancy outcomes.

At each subsequent visit, the blood pressure and urinalysis should be performed and recorded. Urinalysis is often omitted, particularly if the woman fails to bring a sample to the clinic. The importance of screening for proteinuria should be emphasised and samples should always be requested. The full blood count and blood group and antibody screen should be repeated in the third trimester. The fundal height is monitored at each visit although the value of this remains controversial (see Chapter 2). Ultrasound scanning is performed in accordance with local protocols. In some units this will mean a 'routine' anomaly scan at 18–22 weeks of gestation whereas in others, no further scans after the booking visit are performed unless clinically indicated.

Risk assessment

It would be ideal if women at low risk of complications, who would be suitable for midwife/general practitioner antenatal care and who would therefore enjoy less medically intensive care, could be identified early in pregnancy. Similarly, women identified as at high risk at booking could have the resources and skills of the specialist obstetrician concentrated

Table 1.2 Contents of the booking visit
• A thorough history (personal, family, social, medical/surgical, obstetric and drug) should be obtained
• A clinical examination is often omitted but does provide an opportunity to promote health awareness; a full examination is usually unnecessary and this should be adapted to the individual patient's need
• Screening tests for fetal anomaly should be discussed (first trimester nuchal translucency, second trimester biochemical screening, second trimester anomaly scan and fetal karyotyping in selected cases)
• Blood should be taken for full blood count, blood group and antibodies, syphilis screening, rubella antibodies and past or present infection with hepatitis B; counselling for HIV testing should be performed in accordance with local protocols, and screening for haemoglobinopathy should be performed in appropriate ethnic groups
• A cervical smear test can be obtained if indicated
• Maternal height and weight should be recorded, as the body mass index is linked to obstetric and medical problems
• An ultrasound scan will ensure fetal viability, diagnose multiple pregnancy and confirm the gestational age
• Plans can be made for the pattern of antenatal care, the place of delivery, subsequent visits to the clinic; breastfeeding can be promoted

upon them. The concept of risk assessment and formal risk scoring in pregnancy has been summarised by Alexander and Keirse (1989). They evaluated the value of formal risk scoring as screening tests for perinatal mortality, preterm delivery, intrauterine growth restriction and low Apgar score at birth. However, risk scoring performed poorly in identifying women at risk of these conditions (Table 1.3).

Scoring is more effective in parous women than in women pregnant for the first time. The poor predictive value of scoring systems in primigravid women is, at least in part, a result of the choice of risk markers, many of which relate to events in previous pregnancies. This poor predictive value means that the introduction of risk scoring into clinical practice may result in more harm than good. Women who are labelled as being at increased risk of an adverse outcome may suffer unnecessary stress and anxiety and will be exposed to unnecessary investigations and interventions. Scarce resources will be allocated to women who do not need them.

Table 1.3 Formal risk scoring as a screening test in pregnancy

	Sensitivity (%)	Predictive value of an abnormal score (%)	Obstetric population considered at risk (%)
Perinatal mortality	43	6	29
Preterm delivery	36	16	22
Intrauterine growth restriction	41	12	20
Low Apgar score	57	21	12

Cole and McIlwaine (1994) have evaluated risk scoring during pregnancy and have included the outcomes of labour. They demonstrated that, at booking, 96% of primigravidae were considered low risk whereas, by the end of labour, only 39% remained low risk. Forty percent had developed risk factors during pregnancy and a further 17% during labour. Similarly, 74% of multigravidae were categorised as 'low risk' at booking but by the end of labour only 48% remained low risk (24% developed risk factors in pregnancy and 2% in labour).

The evidence indicates that formal risk scoring cannot be relied upon at booking to divide women into high-risk or low-risk groups. Unidentified risk factors will arise during pregnancy and the majority of women will have required some form of obstetric input by the end of their labours. Grant (1995) therefore concludes that, since the majority of obstetric complications will arise in women categorised as low risk, the concept of high-risk and low-risk women in pregnancy and labour should be abandoned. Instead, he proposes that all women are suitable for midwife/general practitioner antenatal care and that locally agreed protocols should be established for the identification, referral and treatment of obstetric complications.

Prepregnancy counselling

For women with specific problems, such as a history of fetal abnormality or a medical condition, such as epilepsy or thrombophilia, prepregnancy care is required. Many of the factors operating to associate such conditions with adverse obstetric outcome can only be addressed adequately before pregnancy. Such care will not only prevent or modify the risk of adverse outcome, but will also allow the woman to make an informed choice as to whether to proceed with a pregnancy, to time it optimally and to obtain appropriate information and advice on the management of

> **RISK FACTORS THAT SHOULD BE IDENTIFIED AT THE BOOKING VISIT**
> - Age less than 16 years or more than 35 years
> - Body mass index over 30 or under 19
> - Medical disorder
> - Past obstetric history
>   previous caesarean section
>   previous stillbirth/neonatal death
>   previous mid-trimester loss or more than three spontaneous miscarriages
>   previous preterm delivery (less than 32 weeks of gestation)
>   previous intrauterine growth restriction
>   previous baby over 4.5 kg
>   previous placental abruption
>   previous severe hypertensive disorder of pregnancy
>   previous shoulder dystocia
>   previous third-stage problem
>   high parity (para greater than four)
> - Family history of insulin-dependent diabetes mellitus, fetal abnormality, genetic or chromosomal abnormality, or thromboembolic disease
> - Booking after 20 weeks of gestation
> - History of drug or alcohol abuse, or social difficulties
> - Multiple pregnancy

any pregnancy. Choices made at this time are preferable to difficult decisions when problems are encountered antenatally.

Examples can help illustrate this problem. Despite good evidence linking folic acid supplementation to the prevention of neural tube defects, few patients on anticonvulsant drugs, associated with a substantially increased risk of neural tube defects, receive folate supplementation prior to conception. As the fetal neural tube closes at seven weeks of gestation, folate supplements initiated at booking beyond seven weeks cannot influence this. Furthermore, the woman on anticonvulsant medication may decide to stop treatment on the diagnosis or confirmation of pregnancy, which itself may be at or beyond seven weeks. In this way, she will expose her fetus to the risk of neural tube defect and herself to the risk of seizures. Seizures carry a threat, not only to her own and her baby's health, but also have implications with regard to her lifestyle: renewed seizure activity could result in her losing her job or driving licence.

References

Alexander, S. and Keirse, M.J.N.C. (1989) 'Formal risk scoring in pregnancy' in: I. Chalmers, M. Enkin and M.J.N.C. Keirse (Eds) *Effective Care in Pregnancy and Childbirth*, pp 345–65. Oxford: Oxford University Press

Cheyne, H., Turnbull, D., Lunan, C.B. *et al.* (1995) Working alongside a midwife-led care unit: what do obstetricians think? *Br J Obstet Gynaecol* **102**, 485–7

Cole, S. and McIlwaine, G. (1994) 'The use of risk factors in predicting possible consequences of changing patterns of care in pregnancy' in: G. Chamberlain and N. Patel (Eds) *The Future of Maternity Services*, pp 65–72. London: RCOG Press

Department of Health (1993) *Changing Childbirth: Report of the Expert Maternity Group*. London: HMSO

Grant, J. (1995) 'The concept of high risk and low risk women in pregnancy' in: CGAG/SCOTMEG Working Group on Maternity Services *Antenatal Care*, pp. 14–19. Edinburgh: Scottish Office National Health Service in Scotland

Howie, P.W., McIlwaine, G. and Florey, C. du V. (1991) *What is Antenatal Care in Scotland?* Edinburgh: Scottish Home and Health Department, Chief Scientist's Office

Munjanja, S.P., Lindmark, G. and Nystrom, L. (1996) Randomised controlled trial of a reduced-visits programme of antenatal care in Harare, Zimbabwe. *Lancet* **348**, 364–9

Scottish Office National Health Service in Scotland (1995) *Antenatal Care*. Edinburgh: CRAG/SCOTMEG Working Group on Maternity Services

Sikorski, J., Wilson, J., Clement, S. *et al.* (1996) A randomised controlled trial comparing two schedules of antenatal visits: the antenatal care project. *BMJ* **312**, 546–53

Tucker, J.S., Hall, M.H., Howie, P.W. *et al.* (1996) Should obstetricians see women with normal pregnancies? A multicentre randomised controlled trial of routine antenatal care by general practitioners and midwives compared with shared care led by obstetricians. *BMJ* **312**, 554–9

Turnbull, D., Holmes, A., Shields, N. *et al.* (1996) Randomised, controlled trial of efficacy of midwife-managed care. *Lancet* **348**, 213–18

2 Assessment of fetal growth and well-being

Introduction

A fetus whose birth weight is low for gestational age is at increased risk of stillbirth, prematurity, intrapartum fetal distress and perinatal morbidity. Such fetuses are at greater risk of impaired neurodevelopment and cerebral palsy in childhood and of other health problems, such as non-insulin-dependent diabetes and hypertension, in adult life. Intrauterine growth restriction (IUGR) encompasses a heterogeneous group of conditions that result in failure of the fetus to achieve its genetic potential for growth prenatally. These conditions include both fetal abnormalities and impaired placental function. The surveillance of fetal growth is one of the main antenatal aims of the obstetrician, midwife and general practitioner. Once identified, the task for the obstetrician is to elucidate whether a small fetus is pathologically small or whether it is 'normal' and genetically small. Thereafter, appropriate monitoring of the pregnancy with timely intervention is required.

Definitions

SIZE

The World Health Organization definition of a small baby is a birth weight of less than 2500 g, but this does not take gestational age into account. Thus, an infant weighing 2500 g at term would be regarded as being small-for-dates, yet an infant of 2500 g at 33 weeks of gestation would be considered appropriately grown. This emphasises the need to use birth weight centile charts in the assessment of fetal growth. The terms, 'small for gestational age' (SGA) and 'small for dates' are statistical definitions of size, when the birth weight lies below an arbitrary centile on charts of birth weight standards, allowing for both age and sex. The centiles most commonly employed are the tenth, fifth or third. If the definition of SGA is a birth weight (or ultrasound-estimated weight) below the tenth centile, then one in ten of the normal population will be included. Even a third-centile definition will still include many normal fetuses and this should be borne in mind when interpreting studies of fetal size and growth. In selecting the appropriate centile, a balance between sensitivity and specificity of the diagnosis is being made (tenth centile is most sensitive and third centile is most specific).

GROWTH

The term 'intrauterine growth restriction' should be reserved for those fetuses with definite evidence that growth has faltered. Growth is a dynamic process of a change in size over time and thus it can only be assessed by serial observation. Fetuses with IUGR may not necessarily be small for dates and *vice versa*. For example, a fetus whose weight falls from the 90th centile to the 30th centile in a short period of time is at greater risk of adverse outcome than a congenitally small fetus that has maintained its size on the fifth centile. 'Genuine' IUGR is attributed to an inadequate supply of nutrition to the fetus by a malfunctioning placenta. Neonatal findings of polycythaemia and hypoglycaemia will suggest whether or not antenatal malnutrition has occurred, while morphometric measurements, such as the ponderal index, skinfold thickness and mid-arm circumference to head circumference, may give an assessment of the nutritional state of the neonate (Figure 2.1).

SYMMETRICAL IUGR

In symmetrical IUGR, the head size and trunk are reduced concomitantly. In most cases, these neonates represent the lower end of the normal range for size. However, some will be small because of an insult that has occurred early in the antenatal period, during the period of general organ growth. The main associated conditions are congenital abnormalities, intrauterine infections and environmental factors.

ASYMMETRICAL IUGR

The fetus responds to an inadequate supply of nutrition by invoking adjustments that maximise the chances of survival. One of these adjustments involves a redistribution of blood flow with more going to the brain, heart and adrenal glands and less going to the liver and kidneys. In consequence, the abdominal girth and the fat stores are reduced more than the head (the 'brain-sparing' effect). This is usually associated with pathology of later onset, such as pre-eclampsia or idiopathic IUGR.

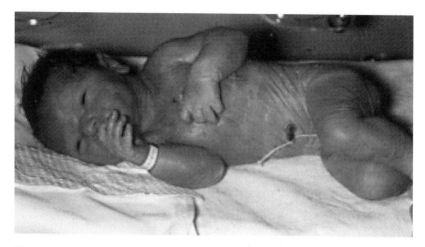

Figure 2.1 Morphometric measurements (see text) indicated that this neonate had suffered from intrauterine growth restriction

Aetiology of IUGR

Numerous factors have been associated with IUGR and the SGA fetus, although actual causes have proven more difficult to identify (Table 2.1). Smoking remains the most important risk factor for IUGR in the general population, with good evidence of a causative role. Roquer *et al.* (1995) have demonstrated that passive smoking is associated with a similar reduction in birth weight as light smoking. Studies investigating the longer-term effects of smoking in pregnancy have demonstrated an association with impaired neurodevelopment at 12–60 months.

IMPAIRED TROPHOBLAST INVASION

Maternal blood supplies the placenta via the uterine arteries, arcuate arteries and the spiral arteries, which, in the nonpregnant state, supply the endometrium. Following implantation, an increase in blood flow to the placental implantation site is required and the spiral arteries undergo profound changes. Trophoblast from the placenta invades these vessels destroying the muscular and elastic layers and replacing them with fibrinoid material and lining the vessels with trophoblast. This process occurs in two waves, the first at the primary implantation time in early pregnancy lasting for several weeks. This reaches the decidual layer of the spiral arteries. The second wave starts around 14–16 weeks of gestation and is completed in approximately four weeks. This wave of invasion, which extends into the vessels as they

Table 2.1 Factors associated with intrauterine growth restriction and the small-for-gestational-age fetus

Maternal medical factors	Maternal behavioural conditions
Chronic hypertension	Smoking
Connective tissue disease	Low booking weight (<50 kg)
Severe chronic infection	Poor nutrition
Diabetes mellitus	Age <16 years or >35 years at delivery
Anaemia	Alcohol
Uterine abnormalities	Drugs
Maternal malignancy	High altitude
Pre-eclampsia	Social deprivation
Thrombophilic defects	
Fetal factors	*Placental factors*
Multiple pregnancy	Impaired trophoblast invasion
Structural abnormality	Partial abruption or infarction
Chromosomal abnormalities	Chorioamnionitis
Intrauterine (congenital) infection	Placental cysts
Inborn errors of metabolism	Placenta praevia

pass through the myometrium, allows the spiral arteries to be invaded by trophoblast to a much greater depth, resulting in a high flow, low pressure circulation in contrast to the high pressure, low flow circulation of the normal nonpregnant situation. This change allows a dramatic increase in blood flow from around 50 ml/min in the first trimester to 500 ml/min at term. This process is inadequate in pre-eclampsia and IUGR, due to placental insufficiency. Where the process fails there is reduced perfusion of the intervillous space. In pre-eclampsia this is associated with a maternal response including hypertension and disturbances of metabolism and coagulation while in IUGR in the absence of pre-eclampsia, there appears to be minimal maternal response with hypertension and metabolic change often being absent. Women with severe or recurrent disease should be screened for an underlying medical condition.

Adverse outcomes associated with IUGR

IUGR is associated with increased perinatal morbidity and mortality, short- and long-term childhood morbidity and mortality, and a range of cardiovascular and metabolic diseases in later life. These are summarised in Table 2.2.

Screening for impaired fetal growth

Much of antenatal care aims to identify IUGR in the general obstetric population. However, tests to assess fetal growth are more sensitive and specific when applied to high-risk women, such as those with a past history of severe IUGR or pre-eclampsia and those with established medical disorders, such as chronic hypertension and systemic lupus erythematosus. The tests perform less well when used to screen low-risk women because of a lack of specificity.

CLINICAL EVALUATION

The detection of women who are at risk of IUGR should begin at the booking antenatal visit. A family history of IUGR or pre-eclampsia should be sought. Previous obstetric history of a growth-restricted fetus should alert the obstetrician to investigate for causes of recurrent IUGR and to ensure that increased monitoring of fetal growth is arranged for the current pregnancy.

Clinical assessment of fetal size by abdominal palpation has been reported to perform poorly in identifying SGA fetuses at delivery, with detection rates between 30% and 50% described in observational studies.

Table 2.2 Problems associated with intrauterine growth restriction	
• Fetal distress (antenatal and intrapartum)	• Hyperbilirubinaemia
	• Intrauterine infection
• Preterm delivery	• Karyotypic abnormality
• Perinatal asphyxia	• Infant mortality
• Stillbirth and neonatal death	• Learning difficulties
• Hypoglycaemia	• Short stature
• Hypocalcaemia	• Cerebral palsy and mental handicap
• Hypothermia	• Adult disease (e.g. hypertension)
• Polycythaemia	

Further, the errors are worse at the extremes of the range when detection is most important. A more quantitative approach is to measure the increase in size of the maternal abdomen, using either the symphysis-fundal height or the measurement of the abdominal girth at the level of the umbilicus. After 20 weeks of gestation, the normal fundal height in centimetres approximates the number of weeks of gestation, with a margin of error several centimetres in both directions. Observational studies have suggested that measurement of the symphysis-fundal height is better than abdominal palpation alone in detecting SGA fetuses, with detection rates of up to 86%. However, one randomised trial found the fundal height measurement to be unhelpful in the detection of low-birth-weight infants, with a pick-up rate of only 28% (Lindhard *et al.* 1990). Further, the detection of low birth weight is not the same as the detection of IUGR. Abdominal girth measurement has not been adequately evaluated.

BIOCHEMICAL TESTS

Biochemical tests that indirectly measure placental function, such as oestriol, human placental lactogen and maternal serum α-fetoprotein (α-FP) have been used as markers of fetal growth. A single unexplained elevated level of maternal serum α-FP in mid-trimester raises the risk of subsequent IUGR five- to ten-fold. The other tests have a low predictive value for adverse outcome and are no longer considered of value in contemporary practice.

ULTRASOUND

Ultrasound scanning is commonly employed in the detection of IUGR and in the subsequent assessment of the fetus. However, a single ultrasound scan performed in the third trimester will not be able to differentiate between SGA and IUGR. Further, the assessment of fetal growth cannot be determined without a pre-existing estimate of gestational age, since the rate of growth for several parameters varies with age. Observational studies indicate that measurements of the abdominal circumference, encompassing the liver, the size of which reflects glycogen storage and nutrition, are better than head measurements, consistent with the brain sparing effect seen in IUGR.

Screening of the low-risk population is usually aimed at detecting the SGA fetus, which is then referred for more intensive surveillance. However, most SGA babies do not have IUGR, while some babies may be of average size but have not fulfilled their growth potential. Controlled trials have demonstrated that routine ultrasound measurement of fetal size in late pregnancy results in an increased rate of unnecessary investigations and intervention, including antenatal hospital admission and induction of labour. Customised growth charts have been designed which take into account several physiological variables that each have a significant independent association with birth weight (Gardosi *et al*. 1995).

PHYSIOLOGICAL VARIABLES HAVING A SIGNIFICANT INDEPENDENT ASSOCIATION WITH BIRTH WEIGHT

- Gestational age
- Fetal gender
- Parity
- Maternal booking weight
- Maternal height
- Ethnic group

Doppler flow velocity waveform analysis of the uteroplacental circulation (maternal uterine arteries) at 18–22 weeks of gestation has been investigated as a screening test for IUGR and pre-eclampsia resulting from placental insufficiency. In a normal situation, a prediastolic notch will be seen in the Doppler waveform. By 22 weeks of gestation the notch will usually have disappeared. This disappearance is thought to be due to the second wave of trophoblast invasion into the maternal circulation which allows the final development of a high flow–low pressure system supplying the placenta (see above). Persistence of the notch suggests that the second wave of trophoblast invasion has not occurred satisfactorily and such pregnancies are considered to be at high risk of growth restriction or pre-eclampsia. The negative predictive value of this test is high, although at present it is restricted to women with known risk factors. One disadvantage of this technique is that the vessels from which signals are obtained are hard to visualise such that repeated measurements from the same site are virtually impossible.

Management of IUGR

QUESTIONS A CLINICIAN SHOULD ASK IN RELATION TO THE IDENTIFICATION AND MANAGEMENT OF IUGR

- Is the baby small?
- Is the growth impaired?
- Is there evidence of placental insufficiency (e.g decreased liquor volume or abnormal umbilical artery Doppler studies)?
- Is there any underlying problem?
- Is the fetus acutely compromised?

Once a diagnosis of IUGR has been confirmed by serial ultrasound scanning, the management will depend upon the gestation of the pregnancy. In late-onset IUGR (after 32 weeks of gestation), antenatal management will involve increased fetal surveillance and delivery if there is any evidence of either acute or chronic fetal compromise. Some would advocate elective delivery after 36 weeks of gestation, while others would continue to monitor fetal well-being until term. Interventions such as stress reduction, stopping smoking, maternal rest and low-dose aspirin are of no proven efficacy. Attempts to improve fetal outcome by nutrient supplements, such as glucose, galactose and amino acids, have not been properly assessed in well-conducted randomised trials and may be potentially harmful to the fetus. Increased monitoring of fetal well-being can usually be performed through daycare units and should involve a measure of acute and chronic fetal condition (see box below). Maternal corticosteroids should be given to improve fetal pulmonary maturity when the diagnosis is made before 36 completed weeks of gestation.

MEASUREMENTS OF FETAL CONDITION
- Acute
  cardiotocography
  fetal breathing movements
  fetal body movements
- Chronic
  liquor volume
  fetal growth

Early-onset IUGR, before 32 weeks of gestation, or symmetric IUGR identified at any gestation, should suggest the possibility of either congenital infection or chromosomal abnormality. A detailed ultrasound scan should be performed to exclude fetal structural abnormality and to screen for markers of karyotypic abnormalities. If a chromosomal problem is suspected, then karyotyping the fetus (via amniocentesis or chorion villus sampling) should be considered, following appropriate counselling of the woman and her partner. Although less commonly performed now, fetal blood sampling for blood gases and investigation of viral infection may be considered. Corticosteroids should be administered and intensive and repeated fetal monitoring undertaken. The management of pregnancies complicated by IUGR is summarised in Table 2.3.

Table 2.3 Antenatal management of pregnancies complicated by intrauterine growth restriction (IUGR)

- Identification and confirmation that the fetus is small for gestational age by serial ultrasound scans; consider whether IUGR or a congenitally small but normal fetus.

- If severe, symmetrical IUGR or gestation <32 weeks of gestation, consider fetal karyotyping and investigation for viral infection.

- Regular fetal monitoring by Doppler ultrasound umbilical artery flow velocity waveform, cardiotocography (CTG) and (modified) biophysical profile scoring.

- If umbilical artery flow velocity waveform and fetal monitoring tests are normal, continue the pregnancy with regular monitoring (twice weekly).

- If the umbilical artery flow velocity waveform is abnormal showing loss of end diastolic flow but other monitoring tests are normal continue with the pregnancy with careful frequent monitoring, at least twice weekly. Should the fetus have reached an adequate gestational age consider delivery.

- Should CTG or biophysical profile show clear abnormalities compatible with hypoxia or the umbilical artery flow velocity waveform shows reversed end diastolic flow proceed to immediate delivery by caesarean section.

Antenatal monitoring of the fetus

It is critically important in the management of IUGR to ensure that the fetal condition is satisfactory. Should there be evidence of fetal compromise at a potentially viable gestational age, delivery, usually by caesarean section, is required. If the fetal condition is satisfactory and tests are indicative of fetal well-being then the pregnancy can be allowed to continue with repeated monitoring until an adequate gestation has been reached. Where there is a concomitant maternal problem such as preeclampsia, delivery may be required in the interests of the mother, regardless of the fetal condition. Several methods of assessing fetal well-being have been described.

FETAL MOVEMENT COUNTING

Since a reduction in fetal movements may precede fetal death by a day or more, fetal movement counting may be of value in assessing fetal well-being. The method most commonly employed in the UK is the Cardiff kick chart, where mothers record the time taken each day to feel ten fetal movements. Women who report a reduction in fetal movements and, particularly, an absence of fetal movements, require a cardiotocograph and/or ultrasound assessment of the fetus to provide reassurance and to ensure fetal well-being. Randomised controlled trials, the largest involving 68 000 women, have been performed to determine whether clinical interventions taken on the basis of fetal movement counting improve fetal outcome. These trials provide no evidence that routine fetal movement counting reduces the incidence of fetal death in late pregnancy. Further, this technique results in more frequent reports of diminished fetal activity, an increased use of other techniques of fetal assessment, more frequent antepartum admission to hospital and an increased incidence of elective delivery without benefit.

BIOCHEMICAL TESTS

Low maternal urinary oestriol excretion has been linked with an increase in perinatal mortality and has therefore been employed as a test of placental function in the assessment of growth-restricted pregnancies. However, this test was not sensitive enough to detect the majority of pregnancies destined to have an adverse outcome, while many women with normal pregnancies falsely appeared to be at risk. Similarly, human placental lactogen measurements have been employed to monitor high-risk pregnancies. These assays are no longer used in clinical practice and have been replaced by biophysical tests.

CARDIOTOCOGRAPHY

Antenatal cardiotocography (CTG) has become widely accepted as the primary method of antenatal fetal monitoring and, in conjunction with ultrasound imaging and Doppler measurements, CTG has replaced biochemical tests. The antenatal CTG is a continuous record of the fetal heart rate obtained via an ultrasound transducer. A further device, the tocodynamometer, detects uterine contractions. The information from these two devices is shown graphically on the CTG. In the antenatal period the uterus is not entirely quiescent and irregular contractions occur which are not usually painful (Braxton-Hicks contractions). The normal fetal heart rate lies between 110 bpm and 160 bpm with a reduction in the fetal heart rate towards the lower end of this range occurring towards term. There are short-term fluctuations in the fetal heart rate due to changes in activity in the autonomic nervous system. This is termed beat-to-beat variability and is normally between 5 and 10 bpm. In addition, accelerations and decelerations can occur.

Accelerations can be defined as an increase in fetal heart rate over baseline by a minimum of 15 bpm for a minimum of 15 seconds. Accelerations on an antenatal CTG are usually seen in conjunction with fetal movements or with a uterine contraction. A reactive (normal) CTG is defined by the presence of two accelerations in a 20-minute period. Reduced variability and the presence of decelerations are abnormal. Variable decelerations can be indicative of reduced amniotic fluid volume with cord compression during fetal movements or contraction. Variable decelerations are irregular in their character. When the umbilical cord is compressed, the venous flow returning to the fetus is impaired, first resulting in reduced venous return to the heart; a transient minor increase in heart rate is occasionally seen. With arterial compression there is a reflex slowing of the heart, which returns to normal as the arterial pressure eases off. There may again be a minor acceleration at the end of the deceleration, as venous return will be impaired for slightly longer than the arterial compression. Late decelerations on an antenatal tracing are uncommon and are usually indicative of hypoxia and a very grave situation for the fetus.

The use of CTG on its own is also termed the non-stress test, as various techniques have been employed in an attempt to stimulate the fetus and look at the resulting fetal behaviour. These have included the oxytocin stress test, where an oxytocin infusion is set up until mild uterine activity occurs; the response of the fetal heart to this can be assessed. Vibroacoustic stimulation has also been used, where a device is held against the mother's abdomen, which produces noise and vibration, when the fetal response can be studied. A physiological test is the nipple-stimulation test, which uses stimulation to the nipples to produce oxytocin that, in turn, can trigger uterine contractility. However, none of these tests is widely used in practice in the UK and the mainstay is cardiotocography without any stress being applied.

Many factors may interfere with the interpretation of the CTG. During fetal rest periods, which may last for more than 30 minutes, normal physiological reduction in heart rate variability may be confused with fetal compromise. Thus, a nonreactive trace must be continued for at least 40 minutes before it can be diagnosed as abnormal. Medications taken by the mother may result in abnormal fetal heart rate patterns while the gestational age of the fetus has a strong influence on the frequency of false positive non-reactive tests.

Initial observational studies suggested a strong correlation between an abnormal CTG and poor fetal outcome and these led to the rapid introduction of the test to clinical practice. Randomised trials were performed in the early 1980s to determine the effects of antenatal CTG monitoring on fetal morbidity and mortality and obstetric intervention.

A meta-analysis of these has concluded that the antenatal CTG has no significant effect on perinatal outcome or interventions such as early elective delivery (Pattison and McCowan 1999). The need for a larger study to address the question of the effect of the antenatal CTG on perinatal mortality was emphasised by these authors.

BIOPHYSICAL PROFILE SCORE

The biophysical profile is a form of fetal assessment based on the concept of the Apgar score used to assess the condition of the neonate (Table 2.4). The profile, which was introduced in the early 1980s, involves an assessment of five variables. These are:

- the non-stress CTG
- ultrasound monitoring of fetal 'breathing' movement
- fetal body movements
- fetal tone (flexion-extension of limbs)
- ultrasound assessment of amniotic fluid volume.

Modifications of the original test have been described, as the equal weighting given to each parameter makes the assessment of all five

Table 2.4 The components of the biophysical profile score

Parameter	Score 2	Score 0
Non-stress CTG	Reactive	Fewer than two accelerations in 40 minutes
Fetal breathing movements	$\geqslant$ 30 seconds in 30 minutes	Less than 30 seconds of fetal breathing in 30 minutes
Fetal body movements	$\geqslant$ 3 movements in 30 minutes	Two or fewer gross body movements in 30 minutes
Fetal tone	One episode of limb flexion	No evidence of fetal movement or flexion
Amniotic fluid volume[a]	Largest cord-free pocket of fluid over 1 cm	Less than 1 cm pocket of fluid

[a]Many obstetricians prefer to use a cut off of 2–3 cm rather than 1 cm in assessing liquor volume

parameters redundant. When the biophysical profile is employed, ultra-sound observation may have to continue for up to 40 minutes before the test can be considered abnormal. The biophysical profile is based on the association between chronic fetal compromise and changes in the fetal heart pattern, decreased fetal body and breathing movements, and redistribution of fetal blood flow resulting in a reduction in perfusion of the fetal kidney and thereby reduced fetal urine production. This, there-fore, is a marker of chronic stress on the fetus with a resultant redistri-bution in organ perfusion favouring the brain and away from the abdominal viscera and fetal kidneys.

A normal score lies between eight and ten and an abnormal score is in the range of nought to four. A score of six would be equivocal and would usually lead to the tests being repeated. Although a biophysical profile may take 30 minutes to complete, in practice in a normal fetus it is quite common for all parameters to have been reached within five or ten minutes in which case the test can be discontinued and classified as normal. As noted above the use of all five parameters is unnecessary. For example, if the CTG is reactive and the liquor volume normal, there is no need to waste resources on assessment of fetal breathing movements. If the liquor volume measurement is reduced and the other parameters are normal, the fetus is still at high risk. In practice, therefore, a modified biophysical profile is more useful; two modified biophysical profiles are a combination of (i) the CTG and liquor volume measurements and (ii) fetal breathing movements, fetal tone, fetal body movements and liquor volume measurements, the former requiring less personnel resources.

In a systematic review of randomised trials conducted to determine whether biophysical-profile scoring is an effective and safe test for the assessment of fetal well-being in high-risk pregnancies, Alfirevic and Neilson (1999) found that, when compared with conventional monitor-ing (usually CTG), biophysical profile testing showed no obvious effect – beneficial or otherwise – on pregnancy outcome. One trial found an increase in the number of inductions of labour following biophysical profiling (Alfirevic and Walkinshaw 1995).

DOPPLER ULTRASOUND

The use of Doppler ultrasound to determine the pattern of waveforms in the umbilical artery has been investigated in more randomised con-trolled trials than any other method of fetal assessment. Fitzgerald and Drumm first described the use of the technique to demonstrate blood velocity waveforms in the fetal umbilical artery in 1977, when it was noted that alterations in fetal umbilical blood flow may occur as an early event in conditions of fetal compromise. Subsequent observational studies demonstrated that the usual umbilical artery waveform had a pattern consistent with a low resistance system, showing forward flow of blood throughout the cardiac cycle. In some high-risk pregnancies, particularly those complicated by IUGR, an absence of flow during diastole was observed (Figure 2.2) and occasionally there was even reversal of flow in the direction of the placenta to the fetus (Figure 2.3). These observational studies indicated that many of the fetuses with abnormal waveforms had a poor outcome.

In recent years, many randomised trials have been performed to assess whether the use of Doppler ultrasound in high-risk pregnancies to determine flow velocity waveforms in the umbilical artery improves subsequent obstetric care and fetal outcome (Neilson and Alfirevic 1999). These have shown that this technique is associated with a 29% reduction in overall perinatal mortality (95% confidence intervals of 50% reduction to no effect). Further, the use of Doppler ultrasound appears to reduce the chances of hospital admission during pregnancy and of elective delivery and induction of labour.

In contrast with its effectiveness in decreasing perinatal mortality in high-risk pregnancies, Doppler ultrasound appears to have little, if any, beneficial effect on pregnancy outcome when used as a screening test in unselected pregnancies.

DELIVERY IN PREGNANCIES COMPLICATED BY IUGR

Timing delivery in these pregnancies depends on balancing the risks to the fetus, if it remains *in utero*, and the hazards from prematurity, which

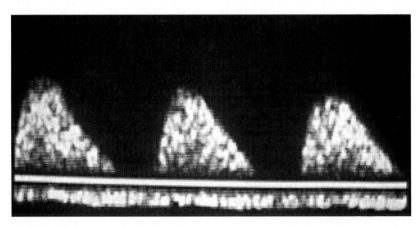

Figure 2.2 Doppler ultrasound waveforms of the fetal umbilical artery, showing absent end diastolic flow

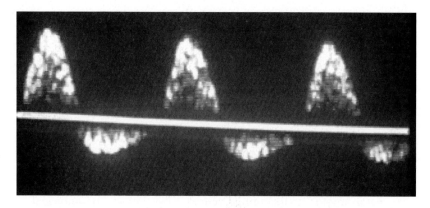

Figure 2.3 Reversed end diastolic flow identified using Doppler ultrasound of the fetal umbilical artery

decrease as the gestation advances. Evidence of fetal compromise on cardiotocography or ultrasound testing is an indication to arrange delivery. If this can safely be delayed for 48 hours, then corticosteroids should be administered (if not already given) at gestations below 36 weeks, to improve neonatal well-being. The mode of delivery will depend upon the gestation of the pregnancy, the condition of the fetus, the state of the cervix and the presentation of the fetus. In the presence of IUGR and oligohydramnios, labour may be poorly tolerated with uterine contractions increasing the risk of birth asphyxia and acidosis, partially due to cord compression

Difficult decisions regarding the timing of delivery may be required when Doppler studies show absent end-diastolic velocities in the umbilical artery with no other serious evidence of immediate compromise at extreme prematurity. These questions are currently being addressed by the Growth Restriction Intervention Trial (GRIT).

The 'large for dates' pregnancy

In a pregnancy that is large for dates it is important to:

- check that the gestation is accurate
- exclude multiple pregnancy if this has not already been done
- assess for the presence of polyhydramnios
- consider the possibility of fetal macrosomia due to gestational or pre-existing diabetes
- exclude underlying fetal abnormality
- exclude uterine fibroids and ovarian cysts.

Polyhydramnios can be defined by an increase in amniotic fluid on ultrasound with a single pool of greater than 10 cm or an amniotic fluid index above the 95th centile (the amniotic fluid index is the sum of the liquor depth in each of the four quadrants of the uterus as assessed on ultrasound scan). The four measurements of cord free pools of amniotic fluid are summated at 34 weeks of gestation; a value of greater than 24 cm would be compatible with polyhydramnios.

CAUSES OF POLYHYDRAMNIOS
- Maternal diabetes
- Multiple pregnancy, particularly monozygotic twins
- Fetal anomaly, including neural tube defect, oesophageal atresia, duodenal atresia
- Fetal hydrops
- Chorioangioma of the placenta

Polyhydramnios can precipitate preterm labour. The presenting part may be ill-fitting and cord prolapse can occur. The increased intrauterine fluid volume also puts the pregnancy at risk of malpresentation and, following delivery, postpartum haemorrhage can occur due to the previous overdistension of the uterus. Administering a non-steroidal anti-inflammatory drug, such as indomethacin, to the mother can restrict the fetal production of liquor or the liquor volume can be controlled by repeated amniocentesis. Indomethacin, however, has adverse effects on the fetus (see Chapter 5), while fluid tends to reaccumulate rapidly following amniocentesis. Overall, management usually reflects the underlying disease, for example in the diabetic woman.

References

Alfirevic, Z. and Neilson, J.P. (1999) Biophysical profile for fetal assessment of high risk pregnancies (Cochrane Review). *The Cochrane Library*, Issue 1. Oxford: Update Software

Alfirevic, Z. and Walkinshaw, S.A. (1995) A randomised controlled trial of simple compared with complex antenatal fetal monitoring after 42 weeks of gestation. *Br J Obstet Gynaecol* **102**, 638–43

Fitzgerald, D.E. and Drumm, J.E. (1977) Non-invasive measurement of the human fetal circulation using ultrasound: a new method. *BMJ* **2**, 1450–1

Gardosi, J.O., Mongelli, J.M. and Mul, T. (1995) Intrauterine growth retardation. *Baillière's Clin Obstet Gynaecol* **9**, 445–63

Lindhard, A., Nielsen, P.V., Mouritsen, L.A. *et al.* (1990) The implications of introducing the symphyseal–fundal height measurement. *Br J Obstet Gynaecol* **97**, 675–80

Neilson, J.P. and Alfirevic, Z. (1999) Doppler ultrasound for fetal assessment in high risk pregnancies (Cochrane Review). *The Cochrane Library*, Issue 1. Oxford: Update Software

Pattison, N. and McCowan, L. (1999) Cardiotocography for antepartum fetal assessment (Cochrane Review). *The Cochrane Library*, Issue 1. Oxford: Update Software

Roquer, J.M., Figueras, J., Botet, F. and Jimenez, R. (1995) Influence on fetal growth of exposure to tobacco smoke during pregnancy. *Acta Paediatr* **84**, 118–21

3 Antepartum haemorrhage

Antepartum haemorrhage, defined as bleeding from the genital tract after 24 weeks of gestation, remains a major cause of perinatal mortality and of maternal and infant morbidity in the developed world. It also remains a major cause of maternal mortality in developing countries. In approximately half of all women presenting with antepartum haemorrhage, a diagnosis of placental abruption or placenta praevia will be made; no firm diagnosis will be made in the other half, which may be due to incidental causes such as cervical pathology.

Placental abruption

Placental abruption, or retroplacental haemorrhage, is the premature separation of a normally implanted placenta from the uterine wall, resulting in haemorrhage before the delivery of the fetus. It occurs in around one in 80 deliveries and the more severe forms are associated with a high degree of perinatal mortality and morbidity. Although maternal mortality is rare, maternal morbidity from haemorrhage, shock, disseminated intravascular coagulation and renal failure is not uncommon. The risk to the fetus depends on the severity of the abruption, gestation, birth weight and the amount of concealed haemorrhage. The perinatal mortality with placental abruption is high and may be over 300 per 1000 (Figure 3.1).

PATHOPHYSIOLOGY AND AETIOLOGY

Abruption arises from haemorrhage into the decidua basalis of the placenta, which results in the formation of haematoma and an increase in hydrostatic pressure leading to separation of the adjacent placenta. As the uterus is still distended with the pregnancy it is unable to contract round the uterine vessels at the placental site, thereby allowing the bleeding to continue. The expanding haematoma can dissect between the fetal membranes, leading to vaginal bleeding. The bleeding, however, may be in whole or in part concealed if the haematoma does not reach the margin of the placenta and cervix so that the blood loss is

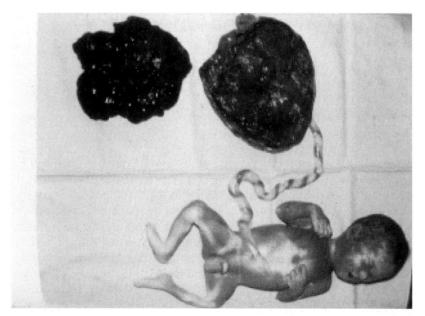

Figure 3.1 Placental abruption is associated with high rates of perinatal mortality; this figure shows a stillborn infant with a large retroplacental clot

revealed. In view of this, the amount of revealed blood loss reflects poorly the degree of haemorrhage, as an enlarged haematoma may be concealed within the uterus. The haematoma may also result in bleeding into the amniotic cavity with subsequent bloodstained liquor being noted when the membranes rupture. Furthermore, the bleeding may infiltrate the myometrium resulting in so-called Couvelaire uterus. This infiltration of blood into the myometrium is associated with sustained uterine contraction, making the uterus feel 'solid' on examination, provoking labour and reducing uteroplacental blood flow with serious compromise to the fetus.

The aetiology of abruption is essentially unknown. It may reflect abnormal placentation as necrosis of the decidua basalis and placental infarcts are often seen in association with abruption. There are many risk factors associated with placental abruption and these are listed in Table 3.1.

Women who give up smoking in pregnancy will reduce their risk of abruption by around a quarter and of stillbirth and neonatal death associated with abruption by around 50% compared with women who continue to smoke. The risk of recurrence of placental abruption in subsequent pregnancies is 7–9%.

Table 3.1 Factors associated with placental abruption

- Maternal age
- Parity
- Deficiency in folic acid
- Low socio-economic status
- Sudden uterine decompression
- Smoking
- Unexplained elevation of maternal serum α-FP in the second trimester
- Severe external trauma
- Uterine abnormality

Traditional obstetric teaching is that there is an aetiological relationship between placental abruption and the hypertensive disorders of pregnancy. However, a causal relationship between hypertension and abruption is controversial, since hypertension can result from the sudden release of vasoactive substances generated from the disturbance created by the abruption itself into the maternal circulation. Furthermore, although there is an association between pre-eclampsia and placental abruption, both of these conditions may arise from abnormal placentation and may be associated with an unexplained elevated maternal serum α-FP in the second trimester. In any event, when hypertension and abruption co-exist perinatal mortality is increased.

CLINICAL PRESENTATION

Placental abruption may occur at any stage of pregnancy. In severe abruption there may be heavy vaginal bleeding or increasing abdominal circumference if the bleeding is concealed and retained within the uterus (Table 3.2). The woman is usually in severe pain and may be in hypovolaemic shock. The uterus may be tender and irritable with palpable contractions or uterine hypertonus often resulting in labour. Fetal distress or intrauterine fetal death may be present. In less severe cases, the diagnosis of placental abruption may not be obvious, particularly if the haemorrhage is largely concealed and it may be misdiagnosed as idiopathic preterm labour. Thus, abruption should be considered in any patient presenting with unexplained vaginal bleeding or possible preterm labour, particularly if fetal distress is present.

Table 3.2 Clinical presentation of placental abruption

- Vaginal bleeding
- Abdominal pain
- Uterine contractility/premature labour
- Uterine tenderness
- Fetal compromise

Placental abruption is a common cause of coagulation failure in pregnancy and the degree of coagulation disturbance tends to correlate with size of abruption and blood loss. Absence of clotting in blood within the vagina may be apparent or there may be bleeding from venepuncture sites or haematuria. The laboratory features of coagulation defect are shown in Table 3.3. Fetomaternal haemorrhage may occur and can result in severe fetal anaemia or fetal death. If the patient is Rh negative, a Kleihauer test should be performed to estimate the volume of fetomaternal haemorrhage, in order to provide sufficient anti-D immunoglobulin.

MANAGEMENT OF PLACENTAL ABRUPTION

In mild placental abruption, the bleeding may settle and the symptoms gradually resolve with satisfactory fetal monitoring and the woman can often be managed as an outpatient. However, she should be reviewed regularly, as the risk of recurrent abruption and preterm labour and associated problems remains increased. The management of moderate or severe placental abruption is to correct the hypovolaemia, deliver the fetus and observe for and correct any coagulation defect that arises. This

Table 3.3 The laboratory features of the coagulopathy in abruption

- Activated partial thromboplastin time prolonged
- Prothrombin time prolonged
- Thrombin time prolonged
- Fibrinogen low
- Platelets low
- Fibrin degradation products increased

requires management in the labour ward with intensive monitoring of both mother and fetus. Guidelines for the management of obstetric haemorrhage have been outlined in the Report on Confidential Enquiries into Maternal Deaths (Drife and Lewis 1998) and are summarised in Table 3.4. Ultrasonography may be of value in confirming fetal viability and presentation since it may be difficult to determine these factors clinically in the presence of uterine hypertonicity.

Table 3.4 Guidelines for the management of massive obstetric haemorrhage

- Staff, including obstetricians, midwives, anaesthetists and porters, should be summoned urgently. Haematologists and blood transfusion staff should be involved at the outset.

- At least two peripheral lines should be set up using cannulae of at least 14 gauge and, if possible, central venous monitoring carried out to guide therapy. An arterial line, if available, is also extremely useful in monitoring the patient's condition. A urinary catheter should be inserted and the urine output carefully recorded.

- Venous blood should be withdrawn for blood grouping and cross-match and coagulation studies. At least six units of blood should be cross-matched initially. Plasma expansion can be provided with human albumin solution or artificial plasma expanders such as polygeline (Haemaccel®). Dextran is contraindicated. In very severe haemorrhage uncross-matched Group O Rh-negative blood may be life saving and two units of blood should be readily available for such emergencies. The blood can be administered rapidly using a pressure cuff and blood warming equipment should be used. Blood filtration will delay transfusion.

- Continuous monitoring of blood pressure, pulse and electrocardiogram should be performed. Blood gas and acid-base status should be assessed regularly.

- Haemoglobin concentration and coagulation status should be monitored regularly. Coagulation tests should be performed to monitor for haemostatic failure, including disseminated intravascular coagulation. Blood products such as fresh frozen plasma or platelets may be required if there is a degree of coagulation failure, which can occur with massive blood loss itself.

- Recourse to procedures such as uterine artery embolisation, internal iliac artery ligation or caesarean hysterectomy should not be left until the patient is moribund and an experienced obstetrician is essential in such cases.

- Consideration should be given to transferring the woman to an intensive care unit.

Management of hypovolaemia

The immediate concern in the haemorrhaging patient is inadequate circulation and priority should be given to restoring the circulating volume. Both clinical assessment and blood pressure measurements are unreliable in estimating the amount of blood loss and fluid replacement should be guided by other means. Central venous pressure monitoring is essential when conducting volume replacement in serious haemorrhage, but the insertion of a central line should be deferred until the results of coagulation studies are known. Large bore cannulae should be sited and blood warming devices and pressure infusion bags should be readily available. However, administration of blood should not be delayed by the use of filters or blood warmers as the priority is to restore volume.

The administration of fresh whole blood will restore the circulation, provide appropriate osmotic and oncotic pressure, carry oxygen and carbon dioxide and restore the depleted essential coagulation factors. Fresh whole blood is now largely unavailable and so packed red cells and plasma expansion are used. However, neither blood nor its individual components are required for the immediate restoration of the circulating volume and administration of crystalloid or colloid solutions may be valuable. The crystalloid solutions that may be given include normal saline or Hartmann's solution but non-salt crystalloids such as 5% dextrose are ineffective. Colloid solutions remain in the circulation longer, an advantage if blood or blood components are not readily available but a disadvantage if fluid overload and pulmonary oedema develop. Dextrans are contraindicated in obstetric haemorrhage since they interfere with platelet function *in vivo* and blood cross-matching *in vitro*. It is recommended that fresh frozen plasma should be given at a rate of one unit for every four to six units of red cells transfused, to replenish clotting factors.

Delivery

When the fetus is alive, a decision regarding the mode of delivery should be made, taking into account the presence or absence of fetal distress, fetal maturity and the degree of haemorrhage. Placental abruption often precipitates rapid labour and vaginal delivery may be possible. Assessment in a severe case of placental abruption should be in an operating theatre set for caesarean section with an anaesthetist present. The examination aims to assess the stage of labour and exclude the alternative or co-existing diagnosis of placenta praevia. If the woman is in labour the fetal membranes should be ruptured as this will advance labour and an electrode applied to the fetal scalp. If fetal distress is present then delivery should be expedited in the form of caesarean section. In the absence of fetal distress, labour, which is usually rapid, should be allowed to progress with continuous monitoring. Clearly, if intrauterine death has already occurred vaginal delivery would be preferred. Abruption also places the patient at risk of severe postpartum haemorrhage.

Management of coagulopathy

Coagulation disorder should always be considered in placental abruption, although defects of clinical significance are rare when the fetus is alive. Massive transfusion itself will cause changes in the coagulation tests, especially prolongation of the prothrombin and partial thromboplastin times, and reduction in the platelet count. Disseminated intravascular coagulation can be identified by prolonged clotting time, reduction in the fibrinogen level and increase in fibrin degradation products (Table 3.3). Fresh frozen plasma should be given to correct the coagulation defects if fibrinogen is very low (4.5 g/l) and bleeding uncontrolled. Replacement of these factors and the decision to transfuse platelets should be undertaken after consultation with a haematologist.

Placenta praevia

Placenta praevia is defined as a placenta that lies wholly or partly within the lower uterine segment. The overall prevalence of the condition is about 0.55% yet it remains an important cause of premature delivery and maternal morbidity. The major cause of mortality and morbidity is haemorrhage as the lower uterine segment forms or the cervix dilates.

CLASSIFICATION

Classification of placenta praevia is important in making management decisions because the incidence of morbidity and mortality in the fetus and mother increases as the grade increases. Many different classifications of placenta praevia have been proposed. Since the condition is most commonly diagnosed on ultrasound scanning, a classification based on the ultrasound findings is appropriate (Table 3.5). Using this classification, types I and II are regarded as minor and types III and IV as major degrees of placenta praevia (Figure 3.2).

AETIOLOGY AND ASSOCIATED FACTORS

Placenta praevia is caused by implantation of the blastocyst low in the uterine cavity. A number of factors are recognised to predispose to the condition. These are outlined in Table 3.6. Placenta praevia is associated with an increased incidence of pregnancy complications including

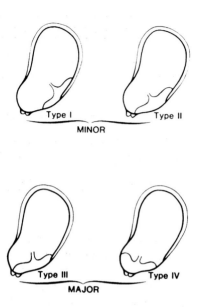

Figure 3.2 This classification of placenta praevia (types I, II, III and IV) is based on the associated ultrasound findings

spontaneous miscarriage, abnormal placentation (including placenta percreta and accreta, particularly with the combination of previous caesarean section and placenta praevia) and fetal malpresentation. Less convincing associations have been made between placenta praevia and the hypertensive complications of pregnancy, fetal growth restriction and fetal congenital abnormalities.

CLINICAL PRESENTATION AND DIAGNOSIS

Classical placenta praevia presents with minor degrees of painless vaginal bleeding in the absence of labour. The bleeds tend to occur at the time of formation of the lower uterine segment, in the first half of the third trimester. Although it is well recognised that some women with placenta praevia do not bleed until the onset of labour, less than 2% of cases of placenta praevia present in this way. Fetal malpresentation or an unstable lie is found in one-third of cases, while a high presenting part is usually present. Vaginal and speculum examination should be avoided in all cases of indeterminate vaginal bleeding until placenta praevia has been excluded, since digital examination in the presence of placenta praevia can initiate life-threatening haemorrhage.

Table 3.5 The classification of placenta praevia based on ultrasound

Type	Description
Type I	The placenta encroaches into the lower uterine segment and lies within 5 cm of the internal cervical os
Type II	The placenta reaches the cervical os but does not cover it
Type III	The placenta covers the cervical os but the placental site is asymmetric with most of the placenta being on one side of the cervical os
Type IV	The placenta is centrally located over the cervical os

The diagnosis of placenta praevia is most commonly made on ultrasound scanning. Up to 26% of placentas are found to be low lying on ultrasound scanning in the early second trimester. However, with the development of the lower segment from 28 weeks of gestation onwards, only 5% of placentas remain low lying at 32 weeks. When transabdominal ultrasonography is employed, differentiation between types of placenta praevia can be difficult, especially in the presence of maternal obesity, overdistension of the bladder, local myometrial thickening, acoustic shadows from fetal parts and posterior localisation. Other techniques including transvaginal ultrasonography and magnetic resonance imaging may facilitate the diagnosis.

Table 3.6 Factors associated with the development of placenta praevia

- Increasing maternal parity
- Advancing maternal age
- Increasing placental size (e.g. in multiple pregnancy)
- Endometrial damage (e.g. previous dilatation and curettage, surgical termination of pregnancy)
- Preterm delivery
- Previous caesarean section
- Cigarette smoking
- Uterine scars and pathology (e.g. myomectomy, endometritis, adenomyosis)
- Placental pathology (e.g. marginal cord insertions and succenturiate lobes)
- Previous placenta praevia

MANAGEMENT

The management of placenta praevia depends upon clinical presentation, severity of bleeding and degree of praevia. In women with minimal vaginal bleeding, expectant management has resulted in substantial improvements in perinatal morbidity and mortality. Expectant management includes the avoidance of vaginal examinations, prolongation of pregnancy until fetal maturity, transfusion support and delivery by caesarean section. In current practice, selected women, usually those who have remained asymptomatic, are permitted to return home as part of expectant management. The clinical course of women with a placenta praevia is unpredictable and many of these women require readmission to hospital for bleeding, although no significant differences in maternal or fetal outcome compared with those kept in hospital have been reported. Where placenta praevia is identified on ultrasonography at 32 weeks of gestation, serial rescanning should be performed to check for resolution of placenta praevia as the lower segment forms. Women with placenta praevia should be commenced on haematinics to maintain a normal haemoglobin, since they are at increased risk of antepartum and postpartum haemorrhage. A Kleihauer test should be performed with every episode of bleeding in rhesus-negative women, and anti-D immunoglobulin administered as required.

The degree of bleeding in placenta praevia is variable, from slight spotting to torrential haemorrhage. Management depends on the degree of haemorrhage and fetal maturity. Delivery should be undertaken:

- when bleeding occurs when the fetus is mature
- where there is associated fetal distress
- when there is persistent haemorrhage threatening maternal health, regardless of fetal maturity or condition.

When bleeding occurs prior to 36 weeks of gestation and the bleeding has been of a minor nature and stops spontaneously then expectant management is warranted. Corticosteroid therapy should be given to promote fetal lung maturity. In torrential haemorrhage, initial management is as described in Table 3.4. In women requiring delivery because of haemorrhage, blood transfusion should commence as soon as possible because further severe haemorrhage is to be expected during caesarean section.

DELIVERY

Caesarean section is the appropriate mode of delivery for all women with type III and IV placenta praevia. Type I and perhaps also type II placenta praevia can be managed conservatively with the possibility of vaginal delivery. If the fetus has not reached a viable gestation, has a lethal abnormality or is dead, then vaginal delivery is appropriate in minor degrees of praevia.

The choice of anaesthetic for caesarean section for placenta praevia remains controversial and should be decided by a senior anaesthetist. If the woman is actively bleeding prior to surgery, general anaesthesia may be preferred as it avoids further lowering of blood pressure, which may occur during regional anaesthesia. Sequential reports on the Confidential Enquiries into Maternal Deaths in the UK have recommended that the operator at a caesarean section for placenta praevia should be senior (consultant or senior registrar grade). The surgical procedure can almost always be performed through a transverse lower uterine segment incision. An anterior placenta will be encountered immediately after incision of the lower segment myometrium and the surgeon must then decide whether to deliver the fetus by cutting directly through the placenta or by reaching round the placenta and separating it off until the membranes are felt. While the first approach is quicker, it may result in severe haemorrhage in the fetus, which can be fatal.

When the placenta is sited posteriorly, there are fewer problems delivering the fetus. Postpartum haemorrhage may occur following delivery of the placenta, owing to an inability of the lower segment to contract efficiently and arrest bleeding from vascular sinuses. This should be anticipated and blood should be readily available before commencing the caesarean section. Furthermore, oxytocics should be administered as soon as the baby is born. In women with a scarred uterus and placenta praevia, the incidence of placenta accreta and severe haemorrhage is increased; such deliveries should be conducted by senior staff.

Bleeding of uncertain origin

In the majority of cases of antepartum haemorrhage, no cause can be demonstrated. The clinical presentation of women in this group is one of painless vaginal bleeding without clinical or ultrasound evidence of placenta praevia. In the initial stages the blood loss is not usually of an extent to cause serious concern. The causes are listed in Table 3.7.

The management of painless antepartum haemorrhage should include an ultrasound scan for placental localisation; if placenta praevia is diagnosed, then further management should be as described above. When the placenta is clearly localised in the upper uterine segment, a speculum examination should be performed to assess the vagina and cervix for a local cause for the bleeding. Once the bleeding has settled and the woman has been observed as an inpatient for 24–48 hours, it may be

Table 3.7 Causes of antepartum haemorrhage of uncertain origin

- Localised placental abruption
- Marginal haemorrhage
- Cervical lesions (e.g. cervical polyp or ectropion, which may cause bleeding, but usually only postcoitally)
- Vaginal lesions
- Excessive show

considered safe to allow her to be managed as an outpatient. The main concern to the fetus in vaginal bleeding of uncertain origin is preterm labour and delivery.

Disseminated intravascular coagulation

Disseminated intravascular coagulation (DIC) occurs where there is gross activation of the coagulation system leading to the generation of fibrinogen, the protein used to seal blood vessels and stop bleeding. Concurrently, there is activation of the fibrinolytic system to break down fibrin. In effect, the fibrinogen generated is rapidly broken down by the active fibrinolytic system. As the coagulation system continues to be activated in an attempt to prevent bleeding, there is gross consumption of coagulation factors and the body is depleted of coagulation factors. There will usually be clinical evidence of bleeding and an underlying clinical problem such as severe pre-eclampsia or abruption. The woman may have spontaneous bleeding from mucus membranes, such as within the mouth or from venesection sites and she may also haemorrhage from surgical wounds.

DIC can be diagnosed by prolongation of the main coagulation tests.

COAGULATION TESTS

Activated Partial Thromboplastin Time
Tests the intrinsic pathway of coagulation containing factors such as Factor XII, Factor XI, Factor VIII and Factor IX

Prothrombin Time
Tests the extrinsic pathway of coagulation, of which the key factor is Factor VII

In addition, it is usual to measure the concentration of fibrinogen (measured either directly or indirectly via the thrombin time), which will be low in DIC. As the fibrin is rapidly broken down, there is an excess amount of fibrin degradation products such as D-dimer. In DIC, platelets are also consumed and the platelet count, normally measured along with a coagulation screen, will fall (Table 3.3). Furthermore, there may be fragmentation of red blood cells in the course of DIC. This is thought to be due to the formation of fibrin mesh within the small blood vessels throughout the body, which breaks up the red cells as they pass through the microcirculation. This is termed microangiopathic haemolytic anaemia and will be seen as a marked reduction in haemoglobin (although this would be present in any case in major haemorrhage); on examination of the blood film, red cell fragments will be seen.

There are many triggers for DIC; those commonly associated with obstetric practice are listed in Table 3.8.

TREATMENT AND PROGNOSIS

The treatment of DIC is, firstly, to deal with the cause. If this is abruption or pre-eclampsia, then the patient requires urgent delivery. Secondly, the coagulation system and haemoglobin levels should be restored by administration of blood products such as fresh frozen plasma and packed red cells.

The prognosis for a patient with severe DIC will vary according to the precipitating factor, the presence of any co-morbid condition, the magnitude of blood loss, severity of the DIC and the extent of other organ involvement. Other organ involvement can occur due to the nature of the intravascular coagulation and the blood loss and it is established that problems such as renal failure or hepatic damage can occur. Once problems such as adult respiratory distress syndrome occur, with associated multi-organ failure, mortality is greater than 50%.

Table 3.8 Obstetric conditions commonly associated with disseminated intravascular coagulation

- Placental abruption
- Major postpartum haemorrhage
- Severe pre-eclampsia
- Amniotic fluid embolus
- Septic shock
- Acute uterine inversion (when associated with major blood loss)

Reference

Drife, J. and Lewis, G. (Eds) (1998) *Why Mothers Die: Confidential Enquiries into Maternal Deaths in the UK 1994–96*. London: The Stationery Office

4 Multiple pregnancy

Prevalence and epidemiology

Twins are traditionally thought to occur in around one in 80 pregnancies, although this is likely to be an underestimate of the true incidence of twin conception. Early pregnancy ultrasound scanning has revealed the phenomenon of the 'vanishing twin', where a twin pregnancy is identified on an initial scan and a subsequent scan shows only a continuing singleton. A twin fetus may perish at any stage of pregnancy. When this happens early in the first trimester, the resulting empty sac will be reabsorbed into the developing placenta and there may be associated vaginal bleeding. If the fetus dies in the second trimester, a fetus papyraceous may be identified at delivery.

There are marked geographical variations in the prevalence of twinning, with a low incidence in countries such as Japan and Taiwan (2–7 per 1000 births), an intermediate incidence in Europe, Australia and the United States (8–20 per 1000 births) and a high incidence in Nigeria, Zimbabwe and Jamaica (more than 20 per 1000 births). These variations are due to the rate of dizygotic twinning, with the rate of monozygotic twinning being fairly constant at 3.5 per 1000 pregnancies world-wide. Twinning rates are higher among black populations compared with whites and Asians. There appears to be a clear genetic component to dizygotic twinning, with the inheritance occurring via the maternal line. Additionally, studies from Italy have indicated that the propensity to dizygotic twinning in the mother could be inherited from both the paternal and maternal sides. Other maternal factors associated with higher rates of dizygotic twinning include multiparity, age 35 to 39 years, increasing maternal height and normal or increased body mass index.

The likelihood of multiple pregnancy is increased in all assisted conception techniques. Ovulation induction resulting in two ova being produced will obviously lead to an increase in dizygotic twinning and a higher than expected frequency of monozygotic twins has also been reported after such treatment. With *in vitro* fertilisation, where two or three embryos may be replaced, there is clearly an increased chance of multiple pregnancy occurring. Although a woman with a history of infertility may view twin pregnancy as a good outcome, higher-order multiple pregnancies are a cause for concern. Hellin's law states that if the prevalence of twin pregnancy was 1: 80 in a population, the incidence of triplets would be 1: 80 squared and that of quadruplets 1: 80 cubed. In the USA, this held true until the mid-1980s, when the incidence of higher-order pregnancies increased markedly as a result of infertility treatment.

Zygosity and chorionicity

Twin pregnancies can be either dizygotic or monozygotic. Dizygotic twins result from the simultaneous fertilisation and development of two ova fertilised by two separate sperm. There is increasing evidence that dizygotic twinning results from excess pituitary gonadotrophin leading to superovulation and it has been shown that women who have previously had a multiple pregnancy have higher levels of the pituitary gonadotrophins, follicle stimulating hormone and luteinising hormone. Monozygotic twins occur following fertilisation of a single ovum by a single sperm and subsequent division of the zygote at various times after conception. In dizygotic twins, the placenta will always be dichorionic, although the layers may be fused together. In monozygotic twinning, the type of placentation will depend upon the timing of division of the fertilised zygote. Very early division (day one to three of development) leads to complete duplication with two fetuses, two chorions and two amnions, which may implant separately or together and fuse in the uterus. This type of monozygotic chorionicity is indistinguishable from dizygotic chorionicity, although the fetuses will, of course, be identical. If division of the fertilised zygote occurs once the inner cell mass is forming (day four to seven of development) each embryo will develop its own amniotic membrane but will share a single chorion; the placenta is described as monochorionic and diamniotic. Division occurring after the amnion has differentiated (day 8–12 of development) will result in monochorionic, monoamniotic monozygotic twins (Figure 4.1). Even later division (from day 12 of development onwards) after formation of the primitive streak, results in incomplete splitting and conjoined twins (Siamese twins).

The antenatal determination of chorionicity by antenatal ultrasound scanning is important since perinatal mortality is increased at least three-fold in monochorionic compared with dichorionic twins. This increased perinatal risk is attributed to fetofetal transfusion syndrome and to twin reversed arterial perfusion sequence. Intrapartum mortality is also high in monoamniotic twins, largely due to cord entanglement.

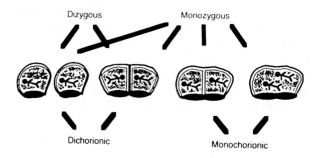

Figure 4.1 In dizygotic twins, the placenta will always be dichorionic; in monozygotic twins, the chorionicity will depend upon the timing of division of the fertilised zygote (see text)

Morbidity is increased in monochorial twins since intrauterine death in one is associated with necrotic neurological and renal lesions in at least 25% of co-twin survivors. Chorionicity can be determined on antenatal ultrasound scanning by:

- counting the placental masses
- sexing the fetuses
- determining the septal thickness
- identifying the 'twin peak' sign, which is formed by a tongue of placental tissue within the base of dichorionic membranes.

Complications of multiple pregnancy

Multiple pregnancy is associated with an increased risk of threatened and actual miscarriage. Congenital abnormalities are more common and women with multiple pregnancy should be offered detailed ultrasound scanning for fetal anomaly in the second trimester. There is increased risk of other pregnancy complications, including hyperemesis, anaemia, disorders of fetal growth, pre-eclampsia and preterm labour (Table 4.1). Premature delivery is the major cause of neonatal death in multiple pregnancy. With an increasing number of fetuses the length of gestation shortens such that the median gestation of twin pregnancy is 245 days, while that for a triplet pregnancy is 231 days and for quads 203 days (Table 4.2). Strategies aimed at preventing preterm delivery have included antenatal uterine activity monitoring, cervical cerclage, prophylactic tocolytic therapy and bed rest. More recently, studies have focused on methods of detecting those multiple pregnancies at increased risk of preterm delivery. These methods have

Table 4.1 Complications of multiple pregnancy

- Exaggerated symptoms of early pregnancy
- Miscarriage
- Loss of twin in early pregnancy
- Fetal abnormality
- Anaemia
- Placenta praevia (due to large placental site)
- Pre-eclampsia
- Preterm labour
- Antepartum haemorrhage
- Intrauterine growth restriction
- Hydramnios
- Twin—twin transfusion
- Postpartum haemorrhage

included transvaginal assessment of cervical length and the detection of the presence of fetal fibronectin in cervical and vaginal secretions.

A particular complication that can occur in monochorionic twinning is twin–twin transfusion syndrome. In this condition the vascular anastamoses between the placentas permit transfusion of blood from a 'donor fetus' to its twin. The donor twin will usually have impaired growth, anaemia and hypovolaemia while the 'recipient' twin may have problems from hypervolaemia, hypertension, polycythaemia and heart failure (Figure 4.2). The recipient twin may also have increased amniotic fluid due to its hypervolaemia, increasing renal perfusion and urine produc-

Table 4.2 Length of gestation in multiple pregnancies (median values)

Pregnancy	Gestation (weeks)
Singleton	40
Twins	35
Triplets	33
Quadruplets	29

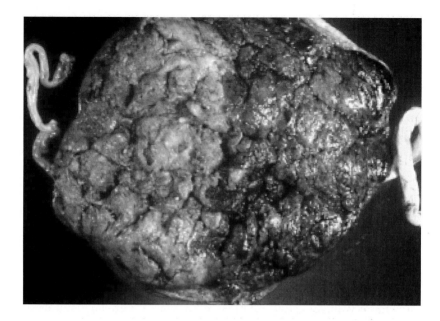

Figure 4.2 Placentas from a pregnancy complicated by twin–twin transfusion syndrome; the 'donor' twin had anaemia and hypovolaemia, while the 'recipient' twin had polycythaemia and hypervolaemia

tion, while the donor twin may have oligohydramnios and appear 'stuck' to the uterine wall or placenta. Although the underlying pathophysiology of twin–twin transfusion syndrome remains incompletely understood, it is well recognised that early onset of the condition in the second trimester, is associated with a high mortality rate for both fetuses. A number of strategies have been proposed for the management of this condition, including laser division of the communicating vascular anastamoses, medical treatment with non-steroidal anti-inflammatory agents, serial reduction amniocentesis and aggressive amnioreduction with rupture of the dividing membrane.

Management of multiple pregnancy

ANTENATAL MANAGEMENT

In most obstetric units, the diagnosis of multiple pregnancy is made in the first trimester on ultrasound scanning at the booking visit. Women who have undergone infertility treatment, who are therefore at higher risk of multiple pregnancy, tend to have several ultrasound scans performed early in pregnancy which may lead to an earlier diagnosis. In units not offering routine booking ultrasound scans, clinical features such as hyperemesis or the presence of a uterus that is considered large for dates should suggest the possibility of multiple pregnancy and such patients should be offered an ultrasound scan as soon as the diagnosis is suspected.

In view of the complications associated with multiple pregnancies, these women are often best managed at a specialist clinic where the problems of twins and, in particular, problems of fetal growth and well-being can be monitored carefully. In the first trimester, the problems of threatened miscarriage and hyperemesis are managed as for singleton pregnancies. The woman should be commenced on prophylactic haematinics (folic acid and iron supplements) to prevent the occurrence of anaemia. She should be advised of the excess risk of preterm labour and told to report to hospital or seek advice from her GP or community midwife if there is any evidence of preterm labour, such as uterine contractions, a show or spontaneous rupture of membranes.

Multiple pregnancies are associated with an increased incidence of congenital abnormalities, including an increased risk of Down syndrome at a younger age in multiple as compared with singleton pregnancies. The risk of one twin with a karyotypic abnormality in a woman aged 31 years is similar to the risk of a 35-year-old woman with a singleton pregnancy. The detection rate for a Down syndrome twin using maternal serum screening (the combination of free β-hCG and α-FP) is less than that for singletons and is not widely available for multiple pregnancy at present. Alternative screening techniques, such as the measurement of fetal nuchal translucency as a marker for aneuploidy, are currently under investigation. Detailed ultrasound anomaly scanning between 18 and 22 weeks should be performed and may identify 'soft markers' of karyotypic abnormalities. Diagnostic testing by means of amniocentesis or chorionic villus sampling may be performed on the basis of maternal age or ultrasound markers. Before these screening and diagnostic tests for fetal abnormality are performed, the woman should be counselled regarding the possibility of abnormalities in one or both fetuses, and should address the issue of termination of the pregnancy, selective feticide or continuation of the pregnancy with no further intervention.

The mother must be monitored carefully for the development of pre-eclampsia, with blood pressure measurements and urine analysis for protein checked at every visit. It is usual to see patients with multiple pregnancy more frequently and, as well as monitoring maternal condition, it is important to monitor fetal growth and well-being. It is important to try to determine whether there is any discrepancy in fetal growth and, in particular, to detect conditions such as twin–twin transfusion and fetal growth disturbance. The only reliable method of assessing fetal growth in multiple pregnancy is by ultrasound. Growth should be determined from abdominal circumference measurements 2–4 weekly from the end of the second trimester to term. If growth is discordant, and this is usually considered if the difference in estimated weight is greater than 20%, then more frequent assessment may be required. When suspected growth restriction occurs in multiple pregnancy, the management is to assess fetal well-being and deliver when the extrauterine environment is less hostile than continuing the pregnancy. As fetal movements perceived by the mother cannot accurately define the well-being of both fetuses, objective assessment of fetal well-being is required and this can be carried out by cardiotocography, biophysical profile scoring and Doppler ultrasound of fetal and umbilical vessels. Cardiotocography can be technically difficult in twins and even more so in higher order pregnancies.

INTRAPARTUM MANAGEMENT

It is generally considered that if a twin pregnancy has any complications, delivery should be by caesarean section. In general, however, the route of delivery is determined by the presentations of the fetuses. The most common arrangement is cephalic–cephalic, which occurs in 41% of twin pregnancies. Cephalic–non-cephalic occurs in 36% and a non-cephalic-first twin occurs in 23%. There is little evidence on which to base the decision regarding the mode of delivery. If the first twin is presenting by the breech, delivery would usually be by caesarean section or if there is a complication such as disturbance in fetal growth or significant pre-eclampsia then caesarean section. Where the leading twin has a cephalic presentation and there are no other complications, labour may be allowed to progress in the anticipation of vaginal delivery. Women with multiple pregnancy should be delivered in a maternity unit with experienced midwifery and obstetric staff in attendance. Appropriate paediatric staff and facilities and an anaesthetist should be available. An operating theatre should be prepared for operative delivery. The woman should have an intravenous line established and a blood transfusion service should be readily available. As operative delivery is often required, epidural anaesthesia should be established early in the course of labour.

Continuous intrapartum monitoring of each fetal heart is essential in multiple pregnancy. Each fetal heart rate should be monitored separately; employing a scalp electrode on the presenting fetus once the membranes have been ruptured can facilitate this. The use of a specific twin monitor, capable of recording both fetal hearts on one trace, helps to ensure that both fetuses are being monitored. Fetal heart rate monitoring of the second twin should continue after delivery of the first fetus since this has been recognised to reduce the perinatal mortality of the second twin. Ultrasonography has an important role in the intrapartum management of multiple pregnancy to confirm the presentation of each of the fetuses and, in preterm labour, to estimate the fetal weights and determine the placental site.

Prior to the onset of labour, Braxton-Hicks contractions occur more frequently in multiple pregnancies than in singletons, presumably due to the increased uterine distension associated with the former. Although the overall duration of labour is similar for singletons and twins, in twin pregnancy the latent phase is shorter and the active phase and second stage are longer. This may be caused by an increased incidence of dysfunctional labour in twin pregnancy, perhaps due to overdistension of the uterus leading to inco-ordinate uterine activity and also, possibly, because malpresentation is more common. An intravenous infusion of oxytocin can be used safely in multiple pregnancy to correct inco-ordinate uterine activity.

MODE OF DELIVERY OF TWINS

As mentioned previously, most of the data relating to twin delivery are retrospective and, at times, anecdotal. In cephalic–cephalic twins, numerous studies have found no difference in perinatal morbidity or mortality rates when vaginal and caesarean section deliveries are compared at any gestation or weight. The evidence regarding the optimal mode of delivery for cephalic–non-cephalic twins is less clear. While the route of delivery appears to have no effect on perinatal morbidity and mortality if the estimated fetal weights are greater than 1500 g, some authors advocate caesarean section if the second twin weighs less than 1500 g. In general, it has become common practice to allow an attempt at vaginal delivery in cephalic–non-cephalic twin pregnancies, regardless of the estimated fetal weights. Breech extraction of second twins weighing more than 1500 g appears to be safe and is associated with fewer complications than intrapartum external cephalic version. When the first twin presents by the breech, the main concern is that of intrapartum twin entanglement; the combination of breech–cephalic twins has the highest perinatal mortality rate. Risk factors for entanglement include:

- intrauterine growth restriction
- antenatal fetal death
- birth weight less than 2000 g

Table 4.3 Types of twin entanglement	
Type	*Result*
Collision	Contact between the two fetuses preventing engagement of either
Impaction	Simultaneous partial engagement of the presenting parts of both twins
Compaction	Simultaneous full engagement of the presenting parts of both twins preventing further descent or disengagement of either twin
Interlocking	Adhesion of the inferior surface of the chin of one twin with that of its sibling. Compaction results if this occurs within the pelvis.

- oligohydramnios
- premature rupture of the fetal membranes.

Four types of twin entanglement have been described (Table 4.3). In view of these risks, together with the proposed risks of vaginal breech delivery of singletons, most clinicians would adopt caesarean section for a presenting breech twin. External cephalic version of the non-vertex presenting twin has been described. Caesarean section is advocated for monoamniotic twins, regardless of their presentations, since twin and cord entanglement are in part responsible for the increased perinatal mortality rate associated with this type of twins.

CONDUCT OF LABOUR

Once the first twin is delivered it is usual to clamp and cut the cord; it is useful to place a ligature round it to identify it as that of the first twin. Abdominal examination is then used to determine the lie and presentation of the second fetus. If the presentation cannot be confirmed then vaginal examination or transabdominal ultrasound will reveal whether this is a head or a breech. Traditionally, the delivery interval between twins has been limited to less than 30 minutes. Continuous fetal heart rate monitoring has improved the outcome for the second twin and, provided this is possible and satisfactory, adherence to a strict delivery interval may not be necessary. Indeed, delayed interval delivery is being increasingly described for very premature multiple pregnancies and appears to be associated with improved outcome for the remaining fetus.

Where the lie of the second twin is other than longitudinal, external version, where the fetus is gently rotated round by pressure on the abdomen, is usually performed to correct the lie to longitudinal.

Occasionally, internal podalic version may be required, where the fetus is grasped by the legs, which are brought down to the vagina to allow breech delivery to ensue. Clearly, in the course of the delivery of a second twin it is important to assess for problems such as cord prolapse. Thus, once the lie and presentation have been confirmed, if the amniotic sac is intact it is usual to rupture the sac and allow the head or breech to descend into the pelvis. Thereafter the delivery is carried out in a routine way for any vaginal cephalic or breech presentation. An oxytocin infusion should be available and used to augment contractions, if necessary, after delivery of the first twin. This also is of value postpartum as the uterus, which has been over-distended during the pregnancy, may not contract normally, resulting in postpartum haemorrhage. Management of the third stage should be active.

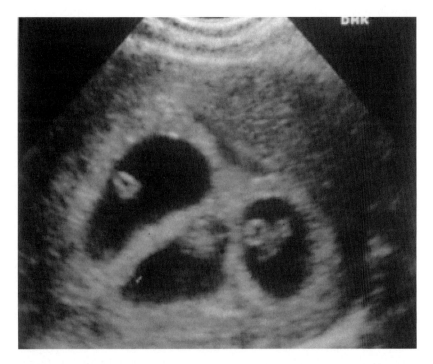

Figure 4.3 Ultrasound scan of triplet pregnancy; higher-order multiple pregnancies are becoming more common as a result of assisted conception techniques

Higher-order multiple pregnancy

Higher-order multiple pregnancies are becoming more common as a result of assisted conception techniques (Figure 4.3). The technique of fetal reduction involves reducing a triplet or higher-order multiple to twins and is most commonly performed around 10 weeks of gestation by the intrathoracic injection of potassium chloride. This technique may be associated with an increased rate of miscarriage but a reduction in the rate of preterm labour. This latter effect should lead to reduced morbidity. However, well-conducted studies with long-term follow-up are required to assess this further.

In view of the significantly increased risk of preterm delivery in these pregnancies, steroids are normally administered from 24 weeks. Triplets and higher-order multiple gestations are probably best delivered by elective caesarean section, since the incidence of malpresentation is higher and intrapartum fetal heart rate monitoring is extremely difficult.

5 Preterm labour

Preterm labour, defined as labour occurring before 37 weeks of gestation, complicates 7–10% of all pregnancies and is responsible for three-quarters of early neonatal deaths in normally formed babies. In those infants who survive preterm delivery, there is a greater incidence of morbid sequelae, including:

- respiratory distress syndrome
- intraventricular haemorrhage (Figure 5.1)
- necrotising enterocolitis
- cerebral palsy
- visual impairment
- hearing loss.

Thirteen million infants are born preterm each year world-wide and the financial and emotional costs to society of this disorder are therefore immense.

PRETERM DELIVERY IS COMMONLY CATEGORISED AS DELIVERY OCCURRING:
- after spontaneous preterm labour (approximately 50% of cases)
- after spontaneous preterm rupture of the fetal membranes (approximately 30% of cases)
- following obstetric intervention aimed at ending the pregnancy for the benefit of either the infant or the mother (approximately 20% of cases)

The prevention of preterm birth is not always indicated, since preterm rupture of the fetal membranes may be complicated by chorioamnionitis and its associated risks, while, in a pregnancy complicated by severe pre-eclampsia or intrauterine growth restriction, delaying the birth may be undesirable for the mother and her infant.

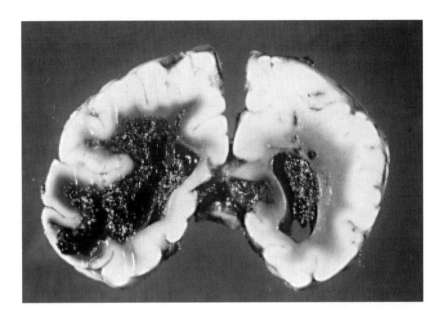

Figure 5.1 Intraventricular haemorrhage is a significant cause of morbidity in infants who survive preterm delivery

Although all births before 37 weeks of gestation are considered premature, births before 32 weeks of gestation account for most neonatal morbidity and mortality. The 20% of preterm births that occur before 32 weeks of gestation and the 10% that occur before 28 weeks of gestation account for 74% and 57% of preterm perinatal mortality, respectively. To investigate increasing survival of infants born preterm with increasing gestational age, Copper *et al.* (1993) investigated over 33 500 infants born preterm in the United States between 1982 and 1986. While no infant survived at or before 22 weeks of gestation, the survival rates increased sharply to approximately 10% at 24 weeks, 77% at 28 weeks, 96% at 32 weeks and over 99% at 36 weeks of gestation. In view of this improved outcome with advancing gestation, the following definitions of premature delivery have been proposed.

Preterm	less than 37 weeks of gestation
Mildly preterm	32–36 weeks of gestation
Very preterm	less than 32 weeks of gestation
Extremely preterm	less than 28 weeks of gestation

Fifteen to twenty percent of extremely preterm infants who survive will have severe neurological impairments or disabilities and approximately half may have more subtle impairments in hearing or intellectual performance.

Prevention of premature birth

ANTENATAL CARE AND SOCIO-ECONOMIC FACTORS

Good antenatal care is important, since it facilitates identification of some of the maternal and fetal conditions that predispose to preterm birth. These factors are listed in Table 5.1. Risk scoring to determine the pattern and intensity of antenatal care has been investigated in several studies of the prevention of prematurity. In general, each of the scoring systems has been able to identify those women with a two-fold increase in the risk of preterm delivery, predominantly on the basis of a prior preterm birth. Unfortunately, risk scoring has resulted in an increased use of interventions with unproven efficacy, with no significant reduction in preterm delivery.

The preterm delivery rate is generally higher in lower socio-economic groups than in high; interventions designed to give social support during pregnancy have unfortunately not been effective in reducing the incidence of preterm delivery.

CERVICAL CERCLAGE

Cervical incompetence is diagnosed in 1:200 to 1:1000 pregnant women on the basis of a history of second-trimester delivery, in the absence of

---

Table 5.1 Risk factors for preterm delivery

- Previous preterm delivery
- Previous cone biopsy
- Previous early pregnancy losses
- Maternal age 30 years or over
- Black race
- High parity
- Multiple pregnancy
- Low prepregnancy weight
- Bleeding after 12 weeks of gestation
- Cervix dilated at 22 weeks

recognisable uterine contractions. Management of women with this condition has traditionally involved the insertion of a circumferential suture (cerclage) in the cervix during future pregnancies. Unfortunately, most women with suspected cervical weakness have histories that make it difficult to differentiate between cervical weakness and early preterm labour. In a randomised study conducted by the Medical Research Council and the Royal College of Obstetricians and Gynaecologists (1993), cervical cerclage resulted in a significant reduction in the rate of preterm birth before 33 weeks of gestation but cerclage was required in 25 women to prevent one preterm birth. Most cerclage operations are performed transvaginally. The transabdominal route is beneficial in treating patients with cervices that are either extremely short, congenitally deformed, deeply lacerated or markedly scarred because of previously failed transvaginal cerclage procedures (Novy 1991) (Figure 5.2).

No satisfactory method of identifying those women who are likely to benefit from cervical cerclage has been found. Several techniques have been proposed to establish the diagnosis of cervical weakness between pregnancies (Table 5.2; for review see Anthony *et al.* 1982).

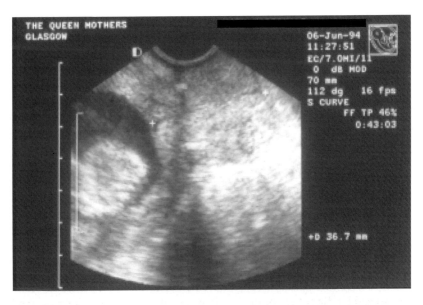

Figure 5.2 Ultrasound scan showing the cervical length (36.7mm) in a woman with an abdominal cervical suture *in situ*

Table 5.2 Techniques proposed to establish the diagnosis of cervical incompetence

- Visual inspection of the cervix to detect a widely gaping cervical os
- Determination of the largest dilator which will pass through the cervix without meeting any resistance
- Radiological hysterography
- Studies with balloons to demonstrate dilatation of the internal os and uterine isthmus
- Use of mechanical force-sensing devices to measure objectively the cervical resistance

BED REST AND HYDRATION

Bed rest and hydration have been employed in women, particularly those with multiple pregnancies, in suspected preterm labour. These interventions have not been demonstrated to be of any benefit and two randomised trials involving twin pregnancies were associated with increased rates of preterm birth. Furthermore, these interventions are associated with other adverse outcomes, including venous thromboembolism and pulmonary oedema.

MONITORING OF UTERINE ACTIVITY

A number of strategies have been tested to determine whether monitoring of uterine activity can reduce the frequency of preterm birth by early identification of women who are developing preterm labour. There is no reduction in preterm births when women are instructed in uterine self-palpation and detection of signs of labour. Electronic monitoring of uterine activity at home, with transmission of the information electronically to a central site, has produced conflicting results. In most trials, this approach has failed to prevent preterm births and is associated with an increased number of unscheduled hospital visits and increased use of tocolytic drugs.

CERVICAL ASSESSMENT

Cervical ripening, which occurs during the last five to six weeks of pregnancy, is defined as an increased softening, effacement and dilatation recognised by digital examination. It is recognised that the frequency of these signs increases as labour approaches, regardless of the gestation of pregnancy. It might therefore be expected that repeated cervical examination would identify those pregnancies at high risk of preterm labour. However, a randomised trial of routine cervical examinations in pregnancy found no benefit from the intervention. Further, vaginal examination increases circulating prostaglandin concentrations and, in one trial, the results suggested that cervical examination increases the risk of premature rupture of the membranes (Lenihan 1984). In an attempt to overcome these potentially deleterious effects of digital examination, ultrasonographic measurement of cervical length to detect premature cervical effacement has been evaluated. It is now recognised that the risk of preterm delivery is inversely proportional to cervical length and that transvaginal ultrasonographic measurement is more accurate than transabdominal assessment (Figure 5.3).

The presence of fetal fibronectin in the cervical or vaginal mucus is a method of identifying women at risk of preterm labour. Fibronectins are a family of widely distributed proteins located in the extracellular ground substance and plasma. Fetal fibronectin is found in amniotic fluid, placental tissue and the extracellular substance of the decidua basalis next to the intervillous space. It is normally found in cervico-

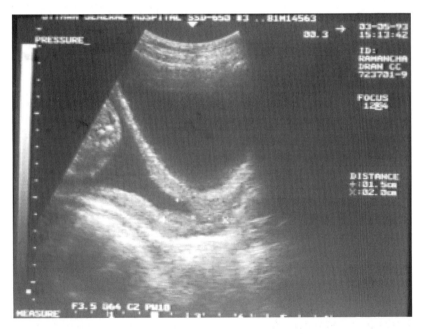

Figure 5.3 Ultrasound scan showing funnelling of the forewaters through the internal cervical os after the application of gentle abdominal pressure; this finding may be associated with cervical weakness

vaginal secretions during the first 20 weeks of gestation. This expression coincides with uterine trophoblastic invasion. Occlusion of the uterine cavity by the amniotic sac leads to the disappearance of fetal fibronectin by about week 20. The molecule is expressed again from about 38 weeks when the process of cervical ripening has begun. The presence of fetal fibronectin after 22 weeks of gestation can be used to identify a group of women at increased risk of preterm birth. Unfortunately, there is a variable time interval between a woman testing positive for fibronectin and the onset of her subsequent labour. Further, false positive results limit its value as a screening test in the asymptomatic population. Fetal fibronectin testing may have a role in differentiating true from threatened preterm labour. Increased concentrations of relaxin in the maternal circulation also show promise as a marker of premature delivery.

NUTRITIONAL INTERVENTIONS

There is an association between low booking weight, poor weight gain during pregnancy and preterm delivery. Various types of nutritional interventions have been studied including counselling and dietary advice, protein supplementation, caloric supplementation and vitamin or mineral supplementation. It remains unclear whether any of these interventions is associated with a reduction in the rate of preterm birth, while the provision of protein supplementation has consistently been associated with adverse outcomes.

PHARMACOLOGICAL APPROACHES

Tocolytic agents are frequently employed by clinicians to prevent uterine contractions in women considered to be at increased risk of preterm delivery. Trials of prophylactic β-adrenergic receptor agonists, both in multiple and singleton pregnancies, have failed to show any reduction in the risk of preterm birth, low birth weight or perinatal mortality. Several randomised trials have evaluated the use of progestogens, including weekly injections of intramuscular 17α-hydroxyprogesterone caproate, in women considered to be at high risk of preterm delivery. A meta-analysis suggests that progestogen administration is associated with a significant reduction in the rate of preterm birth, although there is no decrease in perinatal morbidity or mortality. A recent case report has described the use of the cyclo-oxygenase type-2 selective non-steroidal anti-inflammatory agent, nimesulide, to prevent preterm delivery (Sawdy et al. 1997); prospective randomised trials are required to evaluate further the efficacy and adverse-effect profile of these agents.

TREATMENT OF INFECTION

It is becoming increasingly apparent that substantial numbers of 'idiopathic' preterm labours are associated with subclinical infection of the genital tract. Up to 80% of early preterm births are associated with an intrauterine infection that precedes the rupture of the fetal membranes. Identification of *Trichomonas vaginalis*, *Bacteroides* spp. and *Ureaplasma urealyticum* within the vagina in early pregnancy (10–17 weeks of gestation) increases the risk of preterm labour, preterm, prelabour rupture of the fetal membranes and preterm birth. Similarly, identification of *Gardnerella vaginalis* and *Ureaplasma urealyticum* between 22 and 28 weeks of gestation increases the likelihood of preterm birth. The presence of bacterial vaginosis in vaginal secretions in early pregnancy is associated with late miscarriage and preterm birth, while isolated bacteriuria have also been identified as a risk factor for preterm birth. It is likely that infection contributes to preterm labour and to preterm rupture of the fetal membranes through inflammation and the triggering of the cytokine cascade. There have been many randomised trials of antibiotics for the prevention of preterm labour in asymptomatic women, with disappointing results.

Randomised trials in women at high risk for preterm delivery (usually women with a history of previous preterm delivery) have shown that treatment of bacterial vaginosis with metronidazole, either alone or in combination with erythromycin, may reduce the incidence of subsequent preterm birth. However, these trials have been criticised since, in one, the conclusion was drawn from a subgroup analysis of a small number of women while the other had substantial methodological problems (for review see Brocklehurst 1999). The clinical value of antibiotic therapy in women presenting with preterm labour or preterm prelabour rupture of the membranes (PPROM) is currently being addressed in the ORACLE trial. Recent evidence has demonstrated a link between chorioamnionitis and cerebral palsy; animal studies have shown that chorioamnionitis treated with antibiotics delays delivery but results in white matter lesions in the fetal brain. The ORACLE trial is important since it will evaluate neonatal outcome; in the management of preterm labour, attempts to maintain the fetus in a hostile environment may result in more harm than good.

Preterm prelabour rupture of the fetal membranes

The most common sequel to preterm prelabour rupture of the fetal membranes (PPROM) is preterm labour and delivery, with the interval before delivery being inversely proportional to the gestation at which the membranes rupture. Over 90% of women at term will labour within 24 hours of PPROM compared with less than 50% of preterm women. Fifty percent of women with PPROM will have a latency period of more than one week when PPROM occurs before 26 weeks of gestation. In contrast, almost 50% of PPROM patients will have a latency period of less than four days at a gestational age of 30–34 weeks. The diagnosis of PPROM is therefore extremely important and should be made by sterile speculum examination, with the identification of a pool of fluid within the vagina. A sample of this fluid can be collected to confirm the diagnosis; amniotic fluid is alkaline and contains protein, squames, lanugo hairs and vernix. A high vaginal swab should be taken during the speculum examination and sent for bacteriological culture. Thereafter, an ultrasound scan should be performed to determine the amniotic fluid index, the fetal presentation and the placental site. The woman should be given corticosteroid therapy (see later) and transferred to a unit with tertiary neonatal facilities, if necessary.

The main risks to the mother are preterm labour and delivery, and intrauterine infection. The place of tocolysis in the presence of PPROM is uncertain; certainly in the presence of uterine activity and PPROM, the administration of intravenous betasympathomimetics does not appear to confer any useful benefit. Administration of prophylactic antibiotics in PPROM significantly reduces preterm labour within one week of commencing treatment. The signs and symptoms of infection should be sought (temperature, pulse, vaginal discharge, and abdominal pain) and regular assessments of white cell count and C-reactive protein should be made, especially after the administration of corticosteroids. If there is any indication of intrauterine infection, delivery should be expedited. The risks to the fetus of PPROM include prematurity, infections, cord prolapse, skeletal deformities, pulmonary hypoplasia (Figure 5.4) and an increased perinatal mortality rate.

Diagnosis of preterm labour

Preterm labour is defined as the occurrence of regular uterine activity with associated cervical effacement or dilatation before 37 weeks of gestation. It is often difficult to determine whether a woman is in true or false preterm labour. When preterm labour is diagnosed on the basis of contractions alone, between 30% and 70% will settle spontaneously (false labour). These women are at risk of iatrogenic adverse effects of tocolytic agents administered unnecessarily. Careful diagnosis, with assessment of the cervical state in addition to uterine activity, may improve diagnostic accuracy, although clinical evaluation is hampered by a lack of reproducibility of cervical assessment and difficulty in

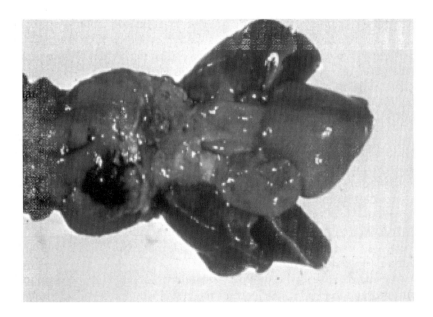

Figure 5.4 In cases of second-trimester preterm premature rupture of the membranes, the fetus is at risk of developing pulmonary hypoplasia; in normal lung development, the lungs should extend to at least the lower cardiac border at post-mortem examination

quantifying the strength of uterine activity. Cervical ultrasonography and biochemical markers, such as fetal fibronectin, may facilitate the clinical assessment. The absence of fetal fibronectin from cervicovaginal secretions in symptomatic women is highly predictive of false labour and tocolytic therapy can probably be withheld in these women. The detection of fibronectin is less reliable in diagnosing true labour but may identify a group of women who are more likely to benefit from tocolysis.

Tocolytic therapy

Numerous pharmacological agents have been employed in an effort to abolish preterm uterine activity. These have included ethanol, diazoxide, magnesium sulphate and progestogens. Of current interest are β-adrenergic receptor agonists, inhibitors of prostaglandin synthesis, calcium channel blockers, oxytocin antagonists and nitric oxide donors. There are certain situations where tocolytic therapy is contraindicated; these are summarised in Table 5.3. The role of antibiotics in the prevention and treatment of preterm labour has already been mentioned. Advocates

Table 5.3 Contraindications to the administration of tocolytic therapy

Absolute	Relative
Fetal death or lethal abnormality	Advanced gestation (? >34 weeks)
Intrauterine infection	Ruptured membranes
Placental abruption	Vaginal bleeding
Suspected fetal compromise	
Maternal condition requiring delivery	

of the link between infection and preterm labour claim that antibiotics treat the underlying cause of the condition rather than suppressing the symptoms, and are therefore fundamentally different from tocolytic therapy. One of the aims of tocolytic therapy is to allow administration of steroids and promote fetal lung maturity.

β-ADRENERGIC RECEPTOR AGONISTS

Isoxuprine was the first betasympathomimetic agent employed in the management of preterm labour in 1961. Since then a variety of betamimetics have been introduced in the hope of developing agents that would have a more selective effect on the uterine smooth muscle and minimal effects on the heart and other body organs.

SOME BETASYMPATHOMIMETIC DRUGS USED IN THE MANAGEMENT OF PRETERM LABOUR
Orciprenaline
Metaproterenol
Salbutamol
Buphenine (nylidrin HCl)
Terbutaline
Ritodrine
Hexoprenaline
Fenoterol

Most controlled trials have investigated the effects of ritodrine. These trials show that intravenous ritodrine can postpone delivery for up to 48 hours, although no decrease in perinatal mortality or severe morbidity has been demonstrated.

betasympathomimetics cause many unwanted effects in both the mother and her fetus. The most commonly observed maternal adverse effects are nausea, vomiting, tachycardia, tremor and palpitations. Women also complain of headache, thirst, restlessness and chest pain. Myocardial ischaemia, arrhythmia and pulmonary oedema are well-recognised complications of betasympathomimetic administration and can be life threatening. Pulmonary oedema, which is more common in multiple pregnancy, results from an increase in plasma renin and anti-diuretic hormone and may be precipitated by administration of excessive intravenous fluids and corticosteroids. The metabolic effects of betasympathomimetics include hyperglycaemia, hypokalaemia and lipolysis. Betasympathomimetics rapidly cross the placenta and stimulate a fetal tachycardia. Hypoglycaemia and hyperinsulinaemia may be observed in the neonate.

PROSTAGLANDIN SYNTHESIS INHIBITORS

The use of agents which inhibit prostaglandin synthesis in the management of preterm labour is logical, considering the evidence indicating that prostaglandins play a crucial role in cervical ripening and in the generation of uterine contractions. Elevated levels of prostaglandin metabolites in plasma and amniotic fluid have been demonstrated during spontaneous labour at term and also in women who deliver preterm. Agents used in the management of preterm labour have included naproxen, flufenamic acid and aspirin, although the most widely used agent has been indomethacin. Indomethacin, which can be administered rectally or orally, reduces the frequency of delivery within 48 hours and within seven to ten days of beginning treatment. The maternal adverse effects of indomethacin include peptic ulceration, gastrointestinal bleeding, thrombocytopenia and allergic reactions. Headache, nausea and dizziness are not uncommon. Gastrointestinal irritation with indomethacin is less common with rectal than with oral administration.

The main concerns regarding the use of indomethacin relate to its effects on the fetus. These effects include prolongation of the bleeding time, constriction of the ductus arteriosus and a reduction in renal function. Long-term administration of indomethacin may influence fetal urine production and result in oligohydramnios. There is no evidence, however, that this agent in preterm labour leads to long-term impairment of renal function in the infant. More recently, indomethacin has been associated with an increased incidence of necrotising enterocolitis (Figure 5.5) and intraventricular haemorrhage in the neonate. Its use should therefore be restricted to short periods and it is unsuitable for use at or after 32 weeks of gestation.

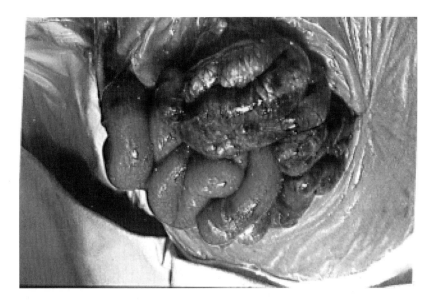

Figure 5.5 Evidence suggests that antenatal indomethacin treatment may increase the incidence of necrotising enterocolitis in the neonate

All prostaglandin synthetase inhibitors act by inhibiting the enzyme cyclo-oxygenase, of which there are two isoforms. Cyclo-oxygenase-1 (COX-1) is the constitutive form of the enzyme whereas cyclo-oxygenase-2 (COX-2) is the inducible form. COX-2 is upregulated during labour in fetal membranes while constitutive fetal prostaglandin synthesis is probably mediated by COX-1. Inhibitors relatively specific to COX-2 would therefore be expected to have the tocolytic effectiveness of indomethacin with fewer adverse effects in the fetus.

CALCIUM CHANNEL BLOCKERS

Calcium channel blockers, such as nifedipine, have become increasingly popular as tocolytic agents subsequent to their use in the management of hypertension in pregnancy. Nifedipine is active orally or sublingually and appears to be as effective in delaying labour as the betasympathomimetics with a more favourable adverse-effect profile. These agents produce vasodilatation and decrease peripheral vascular resistance. Facial flushing and headaches are the most commonly reported maternal adverse effects and, as yet, no serious fetal or neonatal adverse effects have been reported.

OXYTOCIN ANTAGONISTS

While the role of oxytocin in human parturition remains controversial, oxytocin can directly stimulate the myometrial smooth muscle and increase the decidual production of prostaglandins. Further, since oxytocin receptors are primarily located within the myometrium, these agents would be expected to have few systemic adverse effects. The oxytocin antagonist atosiban results in a significantly reduced contraction frequency compared with placebo and has a more favourable adverse-effect profile than that of ritodrine.

NITRIC OXIDE DONORS

In recent years, nitric oxide has been identified as a crucial biological mediator with diverse physiological functions. One of these functions is smooth muscle relaxation and nitric oxide is known to relax the myometrial smooth muscle. Animal studies have suggested that a withdrawal of the relaxant effect of nitric oxide on the uterine muscle is involved in the onset of spontaneous labour. Two observational studies have suggested that the nitric oxide donor glyceryl trinitrate (GTN) may have a tocolytic effect in preterm labour. A multicentre randomised controlled trial was commenced in 1994 to investigate the efficacy of GTN in comparison with ritodrine for the management of preterm labour. Data suggest that GTN is as effective as ritodrine on contractility but just as with betasympathomimetics, no direct benefit in terms of improvement in neonatal morbidity or mortality had been shown. One randomised controlled trial has examined the tocolytic effects of intravenous GTN in the treatment of preterm labour and found that GTN has a higher tocolytic failure rate than magnesium sulphate and is associated with more adverse effects.

Corticosteroids and fetal lung maturity

The use of maternally administered glucocorticoids to improve fetal lung maturity is well established. A 50% reduction in the incidence of respiratory distress syndrome can be expected with benefits seen in infants born between 24 and 36 weeks of gestation. There is evidence from controlled trials that these steroids reduce the incidence of necrotising enterocolitis, periventricular haemorrhage, neonatal death and duration of hospital stay. Preterm rupture of the fetal membranes is not a contraindication to the administration of corticosteroids; these agents remain effective without a definite increase in the rate of infection. The Royal College of Obstetricians and Gynaecologists (1999) has recommended a regimen of two doses of betamethasone 12 mg, given intramuscularly 24 hours apart or four doses of dexamethasone 6 mg given intramuscularly 12 hours apart. The maximum benefit is seen 24 hours after completion of this regimen and lasts for seven days. Repeat courses of steroids can be given but should depend upon continuing assessment of the woman's risk for preterm delivery. Fetal thyroid hormones are important in promoting lung maturation. While maternally administered thyrotrophin-releasing hormone was initially thought to reduce the incidence of respiratory distress syndrome in extreme prematurity, recent trials do not support its use in this situation.

Optimal conditions for delivery

Tocolytic therapy can postpone delivery for up to 48 hours. During this time interval, women thought to be in true preterm labour should receive steroids and be transferred, if necessary, to a tertiary care centre with the specialist neonatal facilities required to manage the expected preterm infant (Figure 5.6). *In utero* transfer reduces the mortality rate and the rate of intraventricular haemorrhage in comparison with neonatal transfer for infants born between 26 and 34 weeks of gestation.

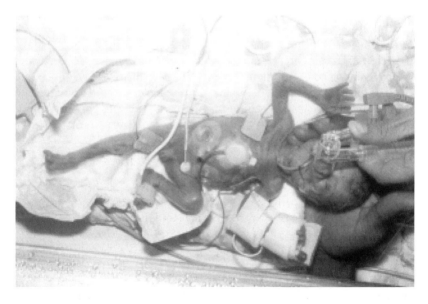

Figure 5.6 Women thought to be in true preterm labour should be transferred to a tertiary-care centre with specialist neonatal facilities

It is important to use the time gained by tocolytic therapy to make an accurate assessment of fetal well-being, presentation and number and to determine the placental position. This will allow decisions to be made regarding the mode of delivery.

Intrapartum management

At the extremes of viability (23–25 weeks of gestation), the mode of delivery and neonatal outcome should be discussed carefully with the parent and paediatricians. Delivery should be conducted by senior and experienced personnel (midwife, obstetrician, paediatrician and anaesthetist). Since the preterm infant is more susceptible to intrapartum hypoxia, continuous fetal heart rate monitoring is generally recommended but only if it has been agreed that it will alter management. The interpretation of the cardiotocograph in extreme prematurity can be complex.

Regarding the mode of delivery, cephalic presentations should be delivered vaginally. The membranes should remain intact as long as possible to prevent excessive fetal compression; 'prophylactic' outlet forceps delivery and elective episiotomy have not been shown to improve the fetal outcome (McNamara and Vintzileos 1997). Delayed cord clamping with the neonate held below the level of the placenta should ideally be undertaken. Between 26 and 32 weeks of gestation, approximately 25% of all fetuses will present by the breech. Delivery of the preterm breech is controversial, although in current practice these infants are usually delivered by caesarean section to avoid traumatic vaginal delivery and, in particular, head entrapment. In this situation, the operative procedure is often difficult because of a poorly formed lower uterine segment and the use of the classical procedure may be necessary. The optimum mode of delivery (caesarean section versus vaginal delivery) remains to be determined.

References

Anthony, G.S., Calder, A.A., MacNaughton, M.C. (1982) Cervical resistance in patients with previous spontaneous mid-trimester abortion. *Br J Obstet Gynaecol* **89**, 1046–9

Brocklehurst, P. (1999) Infection and preterm delivery. *BMJ* **318**, 548–9

Copper, R.L., Goldenberg, R.L., Creasy, R.K. *et al.* (1993) A Multi-center study of preterm birth weight and gestational age-specific neonatal mortality. *Am J Obstet Gynecol* **168**, 78–84

Lenihan, J.P. (1984) Relationship of antepartum pelvic examinations to premature rupture of the membranes. *Obstet Gynecol* **63**, 33–7

McNamara, H.M. and Vintzileos, A.M. (1997) 'The clinical approach to preterm labor' in: M.G. Elder, R.F. Lamont and R. Romero (Eds) *Preterm Labor*, pp. 207–42. Edinburgh: Churchill Livingstone

Medical Research Council/Royal College of Obstetricians and Gynaecologists Working Party on Cervical Cerclage (1993) Final report of the Medical Research Council/RCOG multicentre, randomised trial of cervical cerclage. *Br J Obstet Gynaecol* **100**, 516–23

Novy, M.J. (1991) Transabdominal cervico-isthmic cerclage: a reappraisal 25 years after its introduction. *Am J Obstet Gynecol* **164**, 1635–42

Royal College of Obstetricians and Gynaecologists (1999) *Antenatal Corticosteroids to Prevent Respiratory Distress Syndrome*. London: RCOG Press (Guideline, no. 7)

Sawdy, R., Slater, D., Fisk, N. *et al.* (1997) Use of a cyclo-oxygenase type-2-selective non-steroidal anti-inflammatory agent to prevent preterm delivery. *Lancet* **350**, 265–6

6 Hypertensive disorders in pregnancy

Definitions

HYPERTENSION

During normal pregnancy, blood pressure falls in the first trimester following a decrease in the systemic vascular resistance. On average, the diastolic blood pressure is 15 mmHg lower in the second trimester than before pregnancy. Blood pressure increases in the third trimester to reach prepregnancy levels by term. Hypertension is a clinical sign and the measurement of blood pressure is fundamental in the diagnosis and management of the hypertensive disorders of pregnancy. Blood pressure should be measured with the woman either sitting or lying in the left lateral position (30° tilt) with the sphygmomanometer at the level of her heart. The blood pressure cuff used should depend on the arm circumference, with the bladder length being at least 80% of the circumference. At least two sizes of cuff should be available, with inflation bladders 35 cm and 42 cm wide. In the measurement of the diastolic pressure, Korotkoff phase IV (muffling) is commonly employed, although it is recognised that phase V (disappearance) corresponds more closely to the intra-arterial pressure, is more reproducible and is more closely related to outcome. Blood pressure measurements are often poorly performed and the use of automated devices and ambulatory monitors have been proposed to improve their accuracy.

Hypertension in pregnancy is defined as a pressure greater than 140/90 mmHg. This pressure corresponds approximately to three standard deviations above the mean in early and mid-pregnancy, two standard deviations above the mean from 34 to 37 weeks of gestation and to 1.5 standard deviations above the mean at term. Thus, beyond 30 weeks of gestation, a diastolic blood pressure of 90 mmHg is not necessarily abnormal and may lead to unnecessary intervention. Perinatal mortality increases significantly at diastolic pressures greater than 90 mmHg. Definitions of hypertension based upon a rise in the systolic and diastolic pressures over values in early pregnancy of, for example, 30 mmHg and

15 mmHg, respectively, have been employed. Such definitions will include women who may have a substantial increase in blood pressure, yet the diastolic blood pressure does not reach 90 mmHg. For example, a 17-year-old primigravida with a booking blood pressure of 105/50 mmHg could develop significant hypertension with a blood pressure of 140/85 mmHg at 28 weeks of gestation, which would not meet the definition if a single cut-off is employed. In practice, therefore, it is best to consider both definitions in order not to miss developing pre-eclampsia. When the diastolic pressure exceeds 110 mmHg, this is regarded as severe hypertension and carries a significant risk to the mother, including cerebral haemorrhage.

PROTEINURIA

During pregnancy, up to 300 mg of total protein may be excreted in the urine of healthy women in 24 hours. A urinary protein excretion of >300 mg per 24 hours is considered abnormal. Proteinuria is most commonly detected by the use of reagent strips on routine urinalysis in the outpatient setting. False positive results may occur in up to 25% of women with a 'trace' result and 6% of women with a positive result.

CAUSES OF FALSE POSITIVE RESULTS ON TESTING FOR PROTEINURIA USING REAGENT STRIPS
- Alkaline urine
- Contamination of the urine specimen by:
   chlorhexidine
   ammonia compounds
   vaginal discharge
- Urinary tract infection

To confirm the presence of significant proteinuria, a urinary albumen to creatinine ratio or a 24-hour collection of urine should be obtained and its protein content quantified. Alternatively, the presence of at least (++) of protein should be recorded by reagent strips before significant proteinuria is diagnosed. Proteinuria occurring in the absence of significant hypertension can still be attributable to pre-eclampsia. In practice, the use of reagent strips offers the best utility in pregnancy, particularly in the rapidly progressing case where results of 24-hour urine collections may not be available until after delivery. Objective quantification remains valuable in the overall assessment.

OEDEMA

Although oedema is included in the classic definition of pre-eclampsia, it is of no value as a diagnostic feature since it occurs in up to 80% of all pregnancies. Furthermore, severe pre-eclampsia and eclampsia can occur without oedema and it is of no significance even when associated with hypertension and proteinuria. Oedema may occur in the legs, fingers, face, sacrum or abdominal wall and may be extensive in severe disease.

PREGNANCY-INDUCED HYPERTENSION

Pregnancy-induced hypertension may be defined as elevated blood pressure occurring in a woman in the second half of pregnancy in the absence of proteinuria. The hypertension usually resolves within six weeks of delivery, although the blood pressure can remain elevated for up to three months postnatally. Pregnancy-induced hypertension is associated with a better prognosis for both the fetus and the mother than pre-eclampsia. Pregnancy-induced hypertension can be mild to moderate (diastolic 90–110 mmHg) or severe (diastolic BP greater than 110 mmHg).

PRE-ECLAMPSIA

Pre-eclampsia is a multisystem disorder of unknown aetiology, peculiar to pregnancy and characterised by hypertension, impaired renal function and fluid retention. By definition, it occurs after 20 completed weeks of gestation in a woman who was previously normotensive and with no pre-existing renal disease. Once established, pre-eclampsia progresses at a variable and unpredictable pace until delivery. Both the hypertension and the proteinuria resolve postnatally. The most common presentation is that hypertension occurs first and proteinuria second; however, in 10% of cases the proteinuria is detected first and the hypertension second. In some women, pre-eclampsia presents with a crisis, usually eclampsia or HELLP syndrome (see below).

ECLAMPSIA

Eclampsia is the occurrence of convulsions in pregnancy, not due to a primary neurological problem, in a patient with the signs and symptoms of pre-eclampsia. It is due to cerebral involvement of the disease and is thought to involve vasospasm leading to ischaemia, disruption of the blood–brain barrier and cerebral oedema. Forty-four per cent of cases occur postnatally, 38% in the antepartum period and 18% intrapartum. In over one-third of women, it may be the first obvious manifestation of pre-eclampsia and the woman may be totally asymptomatic or have headache, visual disturbance or epigastric pain. Neurological complications of eclampsia include coma, focal motor deficits and cortical blindness. Cerebral haemorrhage complicates 1–2% of cases.

HELLP SYNDROME

HELLP syndrome (haemolysis, elevated liver enzymes and low platelets) is a serious manifestation occurring in 4–12% of women with pre-eclampsia. Haemolysis reflects microangiopathic haemolytic anaemia and the elevated transaminases reflect liver dysfunction through vascular damage. Thrombocytopenia reflects a coagulation disturbance, although in HELLP syndrome the main coagulation parameters (activated partial thromboplastin time, prothrombin time and thrombin) remain within normal limits. Since elevated blood pressure is not always present at the onset of this condition it may be confused with other conditions causing thrombocytopenia or abnormal liver function tests.

Prevalence of hypertensive disorders in pregnancy

Hypertension complicates 10–15% of all pregnancies and is the most common medical problem encountered in pregnancy. Pre-eclampsia occurs in 4–10% of women in their first pregnancy and remains a major cause of maternal mortality. In the UK, the incidence of eclampsia is 4.9 per 10 000 pregnancies and the death rate for this condition is about 2%. It has been estimated that up to one-quarter of all antenatal admissions to hospital are for hypertensive disorders and it is the most common cause of iatrogenic prematurity. Hypertensive disorders of pregnancy remain one of the main causes of maternal death in the UK. Many risk factors for pre-eclampsia have been identified (Table 6.1). The risk of recurrence of pre-eclampsia is about 5%. This risk is increased in women with an underlying medical disorder and in women with early onset pre-eclampsia or HELLP syndrome.

Aetiology and pathogenesis of pre-eclampsia

The aetiology of pre-eclampsia remains unknown. The primary pathology appears to be defective implantation. The abnormal or damaged placenta releases an as yet unidentified factor that directly or indirectly

Table 6.1 Risk factors associated with pre-eclampsia

- Chronic hypertension
- Multiple pregnancy
- Molar pregnancy
- Renal disease
- Connective tissue disease
- Fetal trisomy 13
- Family history on maternal side
- Congenital and acquired thrombophilia
- Migraine
- Central obesity
- Rhesus isoimmunisation
- Primigravida
- Diabetes
- Age less than 20 years or over 35 years
- Previous severe pre-eclampsia
- Previous severe intrauterine growth restriction

triggers endothelial dysfunction and damage. One possibility is release of a cytokine that can directly stimulate neutrophil activation and/or endothelial dysfunction, producing a vicious circle of vascular damage. Placental biopsy specimens have shown that, in women with pre-eclampsia, the second wave of trophoblast invasion early in the second trimester is incomplete and the maternal spiral arteries adaptation is only about 40% of that in normal pregnancy. In contrast to normal pregnancy, the adrenergic nerve supply to the spiral arteries remains intact. These features mean that the normal, massive increase in uteroplacental perfusion is impaired in the second half of pregnancy, the time when the disease is clinically manifest.

Endothelial cell dysfunction with resultant platelet, neutrophil and coagulation activation appears to be central in the pathogenesis of pre-eclampsia (Table 6.2). This dysfunction is diffuse and may result in widespread circulatory disturbances involving the kidneys and the liver, the cardiovascular and central nervous systems. The cause of endothelial dysfunction remains disputed and numerous theories have been proposed.

Table 6.2 Widespread endothelial dysfunction occurs in pre-eclampsia

- Increased vasoconstriction and reduced plasma volume producing hypertension
- Activation of renin-angiotensin system
- Platelet activation and increased thromboxane A_2 production
- Coagulation activation
- Neutrophil activation
- Increased pro-inflammatory cytokines
- Increased permeability leading to oedema
- Defective endothelial production of nitric oxide and prostacyclin
- Atherogenic lipid profile with hypertriglyceridaemia

Epidemiological evidence suggests that immune mechanisms are involved in the aetiology of pre-eclampsia. Pre-eclampsia is traditionally regarded as a disease of primigravidae. There is a higher level of risk of the disease developing in a first pregnancy than in a second pregnancy. A previously uncomplicated pregnancy to the same partner is associated with a markedly lowered incidence of subsequent pre-eclampsia. A previous miscarriage or termination of pregnancy confers some protection. However, the protective effect of a previously normal pregnancy is lost with a change of partner, suggesting that pre-eclampsia is a disorder of primipaternity rather than primigravidity. Similarly, artificial insemination by donor and oocyte donation are associated with an increased incidence of pre-eclampsia, while the duration of unprotected sexual cohabitation before conception is inversely related to the incidence of pregnancy-induced hypertensive disorders.

Clinical features and diagnosis

Since women with pre-eclampsia may be asymptomatic, the clinical signs of the condition, namely elevated blood pressure and proteinuria, are measured and recorded at each antenatal visit. When symptoms occur, these tend to be non-specific and include rapidly progressive oedema, nausea and vomiting, right upper quadrant abdominal pain, headache and visual disturbances.

Haematological and biochemical investigations are crucial in the diagnosis and management of the hypertensive disorders of pregnancy. The platelet count is a useful marker of disease progression in pre-eclampsia since it tends to fall as the disease advances. However, it has limited

CAUSES OF ENDOTHELIAL DYSFUNCTION

- **Genetic factors**: development of pre-eclampsia may be heredi-tary based on a single recessive gene or a dominant gene with incomplete penetrance. The fetal genotype may influence the penetrance. Genetic factors could govern either defective implantation and/or the maternal response.
- **Placental ischaemia**, resulting in an increased deportation of syncytiotrophoblast microvillous membrane particles into the maternal circulation. These particles have been shown to disrupt endothelial cell function.
- **An immune maladaptation**: an interaction between decid-ual leucocytes and invading cytotrophoblast is required for normal trophoblast invasion and development. Failure of this interaction may result in impaired invasion of spiral arteries by trophoblast and an increased release of cytokines, proteolytic enzymes and free radical species by the decidua which result in endothelial cell dysfunction.
- **An abnormal maternal serum lipid profile**, with reduced anti-oxidant levels and increased free radical generation by the placenta. Central obesity may play a part in this maternal response.
- **Combinations of the above factors**: immune maladaptation, which could have a genetic basis, could promote malinvasion. In turn, this could result in placental ischaemia and release of factor(s) that could stimulate endothelial disturbance and increase free fatty acid release from adipose tissue. The maternal response to this 'stress' may depend on her genotype or phenotype with, for example, women who are insulin resistant developing a greater metabolic disturbance that, in turn, would promote further vascular damage. In any event, the process is complex with many interrelated strands.

value as a screening test in the general nulliparous population because, although the platelet count may be reduced in pre-eclampsia, it usually stays within the normal pregnant range. In more severe cases of pre-eclampsia, haematological changes including haemolytic anaemia can occur, as can coagulation disturbances such as disseminated intravascu-lar coagulation.

An elevated plasma uric acid level occurs before the onset of protein-uria and is a useful marker of disease severity since it increases with disease progression. The normal range for serum uric acid levels is lower during pregnancy than in nonpregnant women. Hence, at 32 weeks of gestation, the upper limit of normal is 0.34 μmol/l and at 36 weeks, 0.39 μmol/l. Raised serum uric acid levels during pregnancy are best regarded as an indicator of impaired renal function and renal blood flow. In women with pre-eclampsia, a rising plasma urea or creatinine indicates a worsening of the disease.

Liver function abnormalities can occur, particularly in severe forms of the disorder. An increase in the enzymes aspartate and alanine transaminase and lactate dehydrogenase reflects alterations in liver perfusion and hepatic congestion. Liver function tests are important in monitoring progression of severe pre-eclampsia and in detecting HELLP syndrome. Where there is major liver involvement, this is often associated with disseminated intravascular coagulation. The main pathological lesions with hepatic involvement in pre-eclampsia are areas of infarction and necrosis. Necrosis occurs in the small blood vessels in the hepatic portal system and also in small branches of the hepatic arteries. Hepatic involvement will be seen in more than 50% of women dying from pre-eclampsia. The hepatic lesion is probably related to activation of the coagulation system and intravascular damage together with lipid accumulation. This situation can progress to liver failure. There may be swelling of the liver resulting in stretching of Glissons's capsule, which in turn may provoke significant pain and vomiting. Haematoma can also occur in the liver where bleeding occurs at sites of infarction. When patients with pre-eclampsia develop right upper quadrant pain, epigastric tenderness and vomiting, it is highly suggestive of liver involvement and immediate delivery should be arranged. Liver rupture carries a high level of maternal mortality.

Severe pre-eclampsia may be complicated by several medical crises:

- cerebral haemorrhage
- eclampsia
- pulmonary oedema
- adult respiratory distress syndrome
- cortical blindness
- renal failure
- hepatic rupture
- HELLP syndrome
- disseminated intravascular coagulation
- placental abruption (cause or consequence?)
- intrauterine fetal death.

The most common causes of maternal death from pre-eclampsia are adult respiratory distress syndrome, cerebral haemorrhage, pulmonary oedema and eclampsia (Table 6.3).

Management of pre-eclampsia

ANTENATAL MANAGEMENT

Prevention of pre-eclampsia

Numerous dietary interventions, including sodium restriction, prophylactic diuretics, calcium supplements and magnesium supplements, have been proposed in the prevention or treatment of pre-eclampsia. None of these interventions has consistently shown any influence on the disease incidence or progression. Supplementation of dietary vitamins C and E and φ-3 unsaturated fatty acids are currently under investigation. The use of low-dose aspirin (75 mg per day) to prevent

Table 6.3 Common causes of maternal death (from Confidential Enquiries into Maternal Deaths)

Cause of death	1985–87	1988–90	1991–93	1994–96
Cerebral				
Intracranial haemorrhage	11	10	5	3
Subarachnoid		2		1
Infarct		2		
Oedema				3
Total	11	14	5	7
Pulmonary				
Adult respiratory distress syndrome	9	9	8	6
Oedema	1	1	3	2
Haemorrhage	1			
Pneumonia	1			1
Total	12	10	11	9
Hepatic				
Necrosis	1	1		
Ruptured liver				2
Liver failure				1
Other	3	2	4	1
Total	4	3	4	4
Overall total	27	27	20	20

pre-eclampsia is based upon the rationale that pre-eclampsia is associated with alterations in the production of prostacyclin and thromboxane, secondary to activation of the clotting system and changes in platelet function. Randomised controlled trials of over 20 000 women have failed to support the routine prophylactic or therapeutic administration of low-dose aspirin. Aspirin may have a prophylactic role in the management of women with a history of severe pre-eclampsia before 30–32 weeks of gestation and it seems likely that these women should begin prophylactic treatment early in the second trimester. It is clear from randomised controlled trials that low-dose aspirin is not associated with adverse maternal or fetal outcome.

Antenatal assessment of women with pre-eclampsia

Much of antenatal care is focused on screening for pre-eclampsia, with regular assessments of blood pressure and urinalysis. The use of maternal uterine artery Doppler studies at 20–24 weeks of gestation has been proposed as a screening test for pre-eclampsia. The value of this technique when applied to low-risk women remains to be determined. Once diagnosed, the severity of pre-eclampsia and rate of progression must be regularly assessed. This will require regular assessment of blood pressure, proteinuria and also laboratory investigations including full blood count and platelet count, together with biochemical assessment of urea, electrolytes and plasma urate. Liver function tests and a coagulation screen should be checked in severe or atypical forms of the disease.

Placental ischaemia occurs in pre-eclampsia. Histologically, there is an atherosclerotic-like lesion in the placental bed with lipid deposition and fibrinoid necrosis. This means that women with pre-eclampsia are at risk of fetal intrauterine growth restriction and management should include tests of fetal well-being. Fetal growth should be assessed by ultrasound scans at fortnightly intervals. The use of Doppler ultrasound assessment of the umbilical artery blood flow is associated with a reduction in perinatal mortality. Fetal well-being can also be assessed using cardiotocography or by measuring the amniotic fluid index. These parameters may be combined with an assessment of fetal breathing movements, fetal movement and fetal tone in the biophysical profile. With early onset pre-eclampsia, iatrogenic preterm delivery may be required and these women should receive corticosteroids to induce fetal lung maturity.

The initial assessment can usually be carried out in a daycare unit, which will allow appropriate assessment of the patient's condition and planning of subsequent management. This assessment should guide whether or not to admit the patient and determine the frequency of maternal and fetal monitoring and need for delivery. The rationale of treatment is to protect the mother and the fetus from the consequences of high blood pressure in order to allow the pregnancy to be prolonged, thus avoiding the problems of prematurity. In many cases continuing outpatient management is appropriate. In pregnancies complicated by hypertension without proteinuria, randomised studies have shown that daycare management can reduce hospital inpatient stay by 60–80% with no detrimental effects on maternal or fetal outcome.

Antihypertensive medication

The purpose of antihypertensive therapy is to protect the mother from the effects of hypertension, including cerebral haemorrhage and eclampsia. Above a mean arterial blood pressure of 125–130 mmHg, there is a loss of maternal cerebral autoregulation. Elevated blood pressure should be treated regardless of its aetiology (in association with pre-eclampsia, pregnancy-induced hypertension or an exacerbation of essential hypertension). By effectively lowering the blood pressure, antihypertensive medication allows the pregnancy to advance and reduces the risk of medical interventions, including hospital admission, caesarean section and premature delivery. However antihypertensive medication does not alter the progress of the disease in pre-eclampsia, nor does it reduce the risk of developing superimposed pre-eclampsia in essential hypertension. When the diastolic blood pressure exceeds 110 mmHg, there is no doubt that treatment is required. When the diastolic blood pressure is between 90 mmHg and 110 mmHg, there is controversy over the management, as blood pressure levels in this range are not usually associated with major hazard to the mother. Thus, some obstetricians will treat if diastolic blood pressure is in excess of 90 mmHg, while others will delay antihypertensive therapy until blood pressure exceeds 110 mmHg diastolic.

A variety of drugs is available for treatment of the hypertension in pregnancy and there is no evidence that any one drug is superior to another (Table 6.4). Since most experience and information is available for methyldopa, this remains the drug of choice in pregnancy. Although safe for mother and fetus, it is associated with minor but troublesome adverse effects, including tiredness, loss of energy, dizziness, depression, flushes, headaches, vomiting and palpitations. Methyldopa is normally started at a dose of 250 mg, two or three times a day, increasing to 500 mg four times a day as required. Alternative medication is labetalol 200 mg three times a day to a maximum of 300 mg four times a day. Beta-blockers are contraindicated in women with asthma and their long-term use, such as in chronic hypertension, is associated with fetal intrauterine growth restriction. If treatment with methyldopa or labetalol fails to control the blood pressure or the woman is unable to tolerate the adverse

Table 6.4 Drugs used for the treatment of hypertension in pregnancy	
Type	*Drug*
Chronic hypertension	Oral methyldopa, a centrally acting α adrenergic inhibitor
	Oral labetalol, a combined α and β adrenergic receptor blocker
	Oral atenolol, a β selective adrenergic receptor blocker
	Oral nifedipine, a calcium channel antagonist
	Oral hydralazine, a direct relaxant of arteriolar smooth muscle
Acute hypertension	Intravenous infusion of labetalol
	Oral or sublingual nifedipine
	Intermittent, intravenous boluses of hydralazine

effects of the first-line agents, nifedipine is added as a second-line drug (10 mg, slow-release preparation twice daily). The adverse effects of nifedipine include headache, facial flushing and oedema. An alternative to nifedipine is oral hydralazine, which can be initiated at a dose of 25 mg three times per day and increased if required to 75 mg four times a day. If a third-line drug is required then labetalol or methyldopa (whichever has not been used as first line) should be employed.

Although generalised fluid retention occurs in pre-eclampsia, the intravascular volume is reduced. Diuretics are therefore contraindicated in pre-eclampsia, except in the treatment of heart failure and pulmonary oedema. Angiotensin-converting enzyme (ACE) inhibitors are contraindicated in pregnancy because of their adverse effects on the fetus. Their use during pregnancy is associated with oligohydramnios, renal failure and hypotension in the fetus. Furthermore, there is a risk of intrauterine death. Women who conceive on an ACE inhibitor should discontinue this treatment in the first trimester.

It is practice at the Glasgow Royal Infirmary to reassess the need for antihypertensive medication in women with chronic hypertension at booking, as patients with chronic hypertension often exhibit the same fall in blood pressure as seen in normal pregnancy. Thus, therapy is often discontinued as blood pressure falls and many of these women become normotensive without treatment. In the second half of pregnancy, antihypertensive treatment with methyldopa or labetalol is initiated as required.

Treatment of fulminating disease

Where blood pressure is uncontrolled, haematological and biochemical investigations are deteriorating or the patient becomes symptomatic, delivery is indicated. The management of the patient with fulminating pre-eclampsia should take place in appropriate surroundings, such as an intensive therapy room on labour ward, and should involve senior obstetricians, anaesthetists and paediatricians working to an agreed protocol. Consideration should be given to blood pressure monitoring using an intra-arterial device and to assessing haemodynamic changes with a central venous pressure or pulmonary arterial line. Haematological and biochemical investigations should be repeated regularly and continuous oxygen saturation monitoring should be performed. The basis of management should be:

- to control blood pressure
- to monitor fluid balance
- to commence seizure prophylaxis
- to arrange delivery.

When blood pressure exceeds 170/110 mmHg, antihypertensive treatment is required to protect the woman from cerebral haemorrhage, cardiac failure, myocardial infarction and placental abruption. Treatment should aim to reduce the blood pressure to less than 160/110 mmHg or mean arterial pressure to less than 125 mmHg. The choice of antihypertensive agents includes labetalol, nifedipine and hydralazine (Table 6.4). The aim is to induce a smooth and sustained fall in blood pressure, since rapid reductions in blood pressure are deleterious to both the mother and her fetus. Many workers advocate plasma volume expansion with 400–500 ml intravenous colloid before commencing parenteral antihypertensive therapy to avoid oliguria and fetal distress; this is best undertaken with concurrent monitoring of the central venous pressure. Fluid balance and renal function must be closely monitored in fulminating pre-eclampsia to prevent iatrogenic complications such as pulmonary oedema, left ventricular failure and adult respiratory distress syndrome. Pulmonary oedema may result from both the over-administration of intravenous fluids and also from the damage to the endothelium of the pulmonary vessels that occurs in pre-eclampsia. Intravenous fluids should be restricted to maintenance crystalloids (no more than 85 ml/hour or urine output in preceding hour plus 30 ml) and urine volumes measured hourly from an indwelling urinary catheter. It is common in severe disease, particularly after delivery, to have transient oliguria, which may last for 24 hours or more.

Seizure prophylaxis is commonly given to women with severe pre-eclampsia to prevent an eclamptic convulsion although, at present, there is no clear evidence that prophylactic anticonvulsant agents prevent the progression from pre-eclampsia to eclampsia. If prophylaxis is administered, the agent of choice is magnesium sulphate, rather than phenytoin or diazepam. Magnesium sulphate is a membrane stabiliser and a vasodilator and therefore reduces cerebral ischaemia and limits any associated neuronal damage. It may also act as a central anti-convulsant in the hippocampus. The treatment regimen for magnesium sulphate is shown in Table 6.5.

INTRAPARTUM MANAGEMENT

Delivery will result in disease regression and is the only cure for pre-eclampsia. For patients with severe disease whose pregnancy is advanced to 34 weeks and beyond, delivery should be arranged. Difficult management decisions have to be made with early onset disease between 24 and 34 weeks of gestation. Postponing delivery may reduce the risks to the fetus of iatrogenic prematurity. However, if the risks to the fetus of remaining *in utero* are greater than the perceived risks of prematurity, delivery should take place if the fetus is considered viable. Likewise, if the risks to the mother from continuation of the pregnancy exceed the risks to the fetus, delivery should be expedited. If the mother has potentially life-threatening disease, she must be delivered regardless of gestation.

When the decision has been made to deliver the fetus, the mode of delivery will depend on the gestation (usually caesarean section at less

---

Table 6.5 Magnesium sulphate for treatment and prophylaxis of seizures

Regimen for the intravenous administration of magnesium sulphate

- Loading dose of 4 g over 5–10 minutes
- Maintenance infusion of 1 g/hour
- Recurrent seizures should be treated with a further bolus of 2 g
- The therapeutic range is 2–4 mmol/l
- Serum magnesium levels can be monitored during treatment

Symptoms and signs of magnesium toxicity

- Loss of deep tendon reflexes
- Respiratory depression and respiratory arrest (treat with calcium gluconate)
- Double vision
- Slurred speech

---

than 36 weeks of gestation), the severity of the disease and the presence or absence of any associated obstetric complication. If a vaginal delivery is attempted, the woman should be regarded as 'high-risk' and her fetus should be monitored closely. When coagulation tests are normal, epidural analgesia should be encouraged since this helps to control the blood pressure. Ergometrine, including Syntometrine® (Alliance), must be avoided for the third stage since it can produce an acute rise in blood pressure. Thus, oxytocin alone is used for prophylaxis of postpartum haemorrhage in the third stage of labour or after caesarean section.

POSTPARTUM MANAGEMENT

Following delivery, the disease process will resolve, although the hypertension and proteinuria may take several weeks to do so. In the immediate postpartum period, the systemic manifestations of the disease may worsen before they begin to settle. The blood pressure may rise in the first week postpartum and a period of oliguria may occur before a diuretic phase. During the period of oliguria, the woman remains at risk of iatrogenic pulmonary oedema and fluid restriction should continue until this has resolved. Diuretics should be employed only when there is evidence of pulmonary oedema. Antihypertensive medication can be withdrawn in the puerperium with blood pressure monitoring undertaken, usually as an outpatient at the daycare unit. Methyldopa is best avoided, where possible, in the postnatal period since it can cause depression. Where the blood pressure remains elevated or severe disease has occurred, the woman should be investigated to exclude an underlying medical condition such as connective tissue disease, thrombophilia or renal disease. Women with a history of essential hypertension can recommence their prepregnancy antihypertensive therapy postnatally. The use of antihypertensive medication, including the angiotensin-converting enzyme inhibitors, is not contraindicated in breastfeeding mothers.

Management of eclampsia

Guidelines for the management of eclampsia have been produced by the Royal College of Obstetricians and Gynaecologists (1996). The woman should be placed in the left lateral position, her airway secured and oxygen administered. Senior medical and midwifery staff should be alerted urgently and intravenous access should be secured. Intravenous magnesium sulphate should be administered to treat the seizures and secondary prophylaxis continued for at least 24 hours after the last seizure (Table 6.5).

Severe hypertension should be controlled with intravenous hydralazine or intravenous labetalol therapy. The woman should be catheterised and strict control of fluid balance maintained as described above. A chest X-ray and arterial blood gases should be performed if pulmonary oedema is suspected. Frequent monitoring of full blood count, coagulation screen, liver function tests and urea and creatinine should be performed. Once the patient is stabilised, fetal well-being can be assessed by cardiotocography and arrangements made for delivery. Vaginal delivery should be considered but caesarean section is likely in primigravid women remote from term with an unfavourable cervix. Cerebral imaging is not considered necessary in uncomplicated eclampsia but is required to exclude haemorrhage in women with focal neurological signs or prolonged coma. After delivery, high dependency care is indicated for at least 24 hours.

Reference

Royal College of Obstetricians and Gynaecologists (1996) *Management of Eclampsia.* London, RCOG Press (RCOG Guideline, no. 10)

7 Common medical disorders in pregnancy

Introduction

In the management of women with medical disorders during pregnancy, a knowledge of the physiological changes of pregnancy is required and considered in the context of the medical condition and its therapy. In planning the management of these cases, there are two key points to be considered:

- the effects of the disorder and its treatment on the pregnancy
- the effects of pregnancy on the disorder and its treatment.

Ideally, the management and assessment of these women should start prior to pregnancy with prepregnancy counselling. This will allow the patient to be counselled with regard to the problems and risks of pregnancy in relation to both her own health and that of the baby and learn how to plan and manage her pregnancy and the risks and hazards associated with it. With this information, she can make informed decisions as to whether or not she wishes to conceive, to avoid pregnancy altogether or delay conception until her medical condition is improved and/or its treatment optimised.

(I) ENDOCRINE DISORDERS

Diabetes

PHYSIOLOGICAL CHANGES DURING PREGNANCY

Pregnancy is a state of relative insulin resistance. Hormones secreted largely by the placenta, which include human placental lactogen, glucagon and cortisol, antagonise the effects of insulin. As a result, postprandial glucose levels are increased compared to the nonpregnant state. To compensate for these effects, the production of insulin is doubled during normal pregnancy, while the insulin requirements of insulin dependent diabetic women are substantially increased. Fasting glucose levels are decreased during pregnancy compared to the nonpregnant state. Finally, the ability of the kidneys to handle glucose during pregnancy is altered and glycosuria is a common finding in normal pregnancy.

BACKGROUND

Insulin-dependent diabetes mellitus (IDDM, type 1) affects about 0.5% of the UK population and tends to present in children or young adults who are of normal weight. In contrast, non-insulin-dependent diabetes (NIDDM, type 2) occurs in an older and often overweight population. Both IDDM and NIDDM may present with the 'classical' symptoms of polyuria, polydipsia and weight loss, or with complications of the disease, including infection, visual disturbance or microvascular disease. In the presence of symptoms, the diagnosis of diabetes is made when a random blood glucose is $\geqslant 11.1$ mmol/l or a fasting blood glucose is $\geqslant 7.0$ mmol/l. As outlined above, pregnancy has profound effects on diabetic control and insulin requirements. Although there is a general agreement that IDDM has many adverse effects on pregnancy, the diagnosis, significance and management of lesser degrees of hyperglycaemia ('impaired glucose tolerance' and 'gestational diabetes') remain controversial.

Effect of pregnancy on diabetes

Women with IDDM require increased doses of insulin during pregnancy. Often by term, insulin requirements are two-fold greater than prepregnancy. As a result of tighter glucose control, episodes of hypoglycaemia are more common during pregnancy. Ketoacidosis is uncommon in pregnancy but should be considered in pregnancies complicated by hyperemesis or infection. Diabetic control may be markedly disturbed when corticosteroids or betasympathomimetics are employed during pregnancy. Most women with nephropathy will experience no deterioration in renal function during pregnancy, although some women experience a significant deterioration that does not always improve postnatally. Pregnancy appears to cause a worsening of diabetic retinopathy and regular ophthalmological examination should be made during any diabetic pregnancy.

Effect of diabetes on pregnancy

Diabetes in pregnancy is associated with an increased incidence of complications (Table 7.1). There is an increased risk of congenital abnormality, up to three-fold greater than in non-diabetic pregnancies, particularly cardiac, renal and neural tube defects. Sacral agenesis, which is specific to diabetic pregnancies, is rare. This increased risk of abnormality is related to maternal hyperglycaemia during embryogenesis and

Table 7.1 Adverse effects of diabetes on pregnancy

- Congenital abnormality
- Miscarriage
- Pre-eclampsia
- Unexplained intrauterine death (? related to fetal metabolic disturbance resulting in acidosis)
- Intrauterine growth restriction (diabetics with microvascular disease)
- Fetal macrosomia
    — shoulder dystocia
    — polyhydramnios
    — increased caesarean section rate
    — increased risk of metabolic disturbance in the fetus
- Increased perinatal and neonatal mortality rates
- Infection

may be correlated with glycosylated haemoglobin. This emphasises the importance of prepregnancy care to obtain optimal glycaemic control prior to conception. Miscarriage is more common in poorly controlled diabetics. Disturbances in fetal growth can occur. This includes macrosomia (Figure 7.1), which is more common in poorly controlled disease but can occur in pregnancies with good glycaemic control, and intrauterine growth restriction, which is associated with women with microvascular disease.

Diabetic pregnancies are associated with increased perinatal and neonatal mortality rates. With improvements in management and advances in neonatal care, the perinatal mortality in pregnancy complicated by diabetes has been reduced ten-fold in the past four decades and some specialist centres claim perinatal mortality rates close to those of non-diabetic women. However, the risk of unexplained intrauterine death, particularly in the late third trimester, remains. Diabetes will also place the mother at increased risk of antenatal problems such as pre-eclampsia and infections particularly urinary tract infection and vaginal candidiasis.

MANAGEMENT OF DIABETIC PREGNANCY

Prepregnancy

Ideally, management should start before pregnancy, when the patient should receive advice about the importance of good glycaemic control

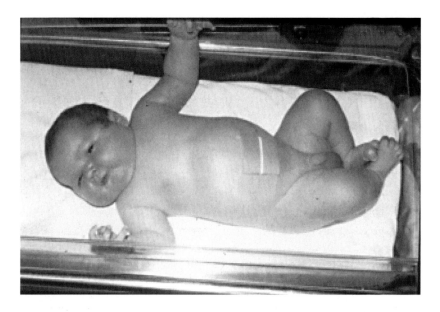

Figure 7.1 Fetal macrosomia is more common in poorly controlled diabetes but can occur in pregnancies with good glycaemic control

prior to and during the early weeks of pregnancy to avoid or minimise the risk of fetal abnormality. Folic acid supplements may also be of value in preventing neural tube defects. Diabetic women should be made aware of the problems that can occur during pregnancy and the need for increased vigilance, both in maternal and fetal interests. The importance of early ultrasound to confirm dates and viability and the availability of prenatal diagnostic tests should be discussed. Prepregnancy counselling provides the opportunity to assess the severity of associated vascular complications, nephropathy or hypertension. Women with diabetes can be reassured that there is no evidence that diabetes complicating pregnancy has any long-term adverse effects on their children's intelligence or development. Less than 2% of their children will develop juvenile diabetes.

Antenatal management

Diabetic women should receive their antenatal care at clinics managed jointly by obstetricians and physicians with a special interest in this disorder. This allows the involvement of other healthcare workers, including dieticians and specialist midwives. One of the most important aspects of antenatal care is to achieve optimal glycaemic control throughout the pregnancy, with a target blood sugar concentration of 4–6 mmol/l before meals and < 7.5 mmol/l postprandially. Glycosylated haemoglobin measurements are useful to assess the degree of diabetic control. Insulin therapy will require to be adjusted, usually switching from twice daily insulin to four-times daily administration. This usually takes the form of short-acting insulin preprandially before breakfast, lunch and dinner with an intermediate-acting insulin at night-time.

Some women will require admission to the antenatal wards to alter their insulin regimen in the first trimester. Those who remain as outpatients should closely monitor their blood glucose levels using glucose oxidase strips and glucose meters. The use of home monitoring significantly reduces the time that these women spend in hospital without affecting pregnancy outcomes. Hypoglycaemia is a relatively common occurrence, especially when tight diabetic control is the aim, and it is important that both she and her partner are aware of this risk and how to remedy the situation using intramuscular glucagon injections when she is unable to eat. Dietary advice is important to ensure that the woman adheres to high-fibre, low-sugar, low-fat foods.

Those women with diabetic nephropathy should have serial assessments of renal function and their urine should be examined regularly for infection. Ophthalmological examination should be performed in each trimester, especially in women who have had diabetes for more than ten years. Proteinuria and blood pressure measurements should be performed regularly.

In view of the increased risk of fetal abnormalities, these women should be offered second-trimester biochemical screening (Figure 7.2); detailed ultrasound scanning should be performed at 18–20 weeks of gestation. The assessment of maternal uterine artery waveforms by Doppler ultrasound in the prediction of hypertensive disorders requires further evaluation, but clearly may be of value in diabetic pregnancy. In the late second and third trimesters, fortnightly assessment of fetal growth velocity and liquor volume by ultrasound may detect macrosomia, intrauterine growth restriction or polyhydramnios. Where there is any evidence of growth disturbance, assessment of fetal well-being should be carried out by way of cardiotocography, biophysical profiles and assessment of umbilical artery waveforms by Doppler ultrasound.

Intrapartum management

In view of the risk of unexplained intrauterine death, particularly after 36 weeks of gestation, elective preterm delivery has been advocated. Studies have shown that this strategy does not reduce the perinatal mortality while exposing the neonate to the risks of the respiratory distress syndrome. Current management is to allow well-controlled diabetics to continue until term and to aim for vaginal delivery. Both elective and emergency caesarean section rates are higher in these women and

PRENATAL SCREENING ASSAY REPORT

FROM: DUNCAN GUTHRIE INST. OF MEDICAL GENETICS
YORKHILL, GLASGOW G3 8SJ
Tel: 0141-201 0372

Date Sample Taken: 12-09-00

Lab. Ref. No.: 654321

Surname: ANYBODY	Hospital: GLASGOW ROYAL MATERNITY
Forename: JANE	Address: HOSPITAL
Address: 1 ANY ROAD	ROTTENROW
ANYTOWN	GLASGOW
	Hospital No.: 654321
Weight: 70.0 Kg. Height: 1.64 m.	Clinic/Ward:
Date of Birth: 01-06-75	Consultant

Previous Serum Report Number   None

	By Dates	Ultrasound
L.M.P. 19-05-00 Certain Gestation	16+4	16+4

Previous History of Neural Tube Defect   No

Complication of this Pregnancy   Insulin Dep Diabetic

Remarks

Serum AFP result: 84.5   kU/l   Weight adjusted AFP = 2.79 MOM

Serum hCG result: 30   IU/ml   Weight adjusted HCG = 1.08 MOM

Comment   AFP value elevated for the earliest stated gestation. Please check AFP guide-lines below.

The AFP and HCG results at maternal age 25 years, 104 days give a combined risk of Down's syndrome at mid trimester of less than 1:220, which falls within the LOW RISK group (see graph).

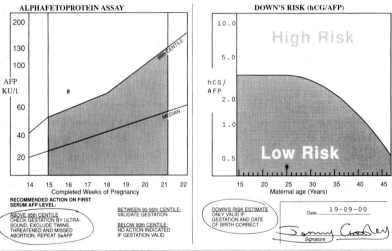

Figure 7.2 In view of the increased risk of fetal abnormalities in women with diabetes, it is Glasgow Royal Infirmary practice to offer second-trimester biochemical screening and detailed ultrasound scanning; this serum screening report shows an elevated maternal serum α-fetoprotein level

are partly explained by the associated higher median birth weight for gestation. The main hazard of vaginal delivery in women with diabetes is of shoulder dystocia with a macrosomic fetus. The risks of shoulder dystocia and brachial plexus injury are greater in infants of diabetic mothers than similarly sized infants of non-diabetic mothers.

During labour, glycaemic control is achieved by an intravenous infusion of 5–10% glucose/saline administered at an initial rate of 100 ml/hour in conjunction with an intravenous infusion of soluble insulin at an initial dose of one unit/hour, titrating this against hourly blood glucose measurements. The target glucose during labour is 4–7 mmol/l and hypoglycaemia should be avoided. If a caesarean section is performed, prophylactic antibiotics should be given, in view of the excess risk of infection with diabetes in pregnancy. Following delivery of the placenta, the intravenous insulin infusion should be discontinued, and the prepregnancy insulin regimen recommenced. This may need to be altered to accommodate breastfeeding. The neonate will be at excess risk of problems such as respiratory distress syndrome, hypoglycaemia, polycythaemia and neonatal jaundice.

GESTATIONAL DIABETES AND IMPAIRED GLUCOSE TOLERANCE

Diabetes can present for the first time in pregnancy but more often this is a gestation-related phenomenon. The diagnosis and importance of gestational diabetes are controversial. Since carbohydrate intolerance and a degree of insulin resistance are not unusual during pregnancy, any woman who cannot compensate sufficiently for these will develop an abnormal glucose tolerance test. Gestational diabetes should be suspected in women with a macrosomic fetus, polyhydramnios, persistent glycosuria or recurrent infections. Consideration should also be given to women with a strong family history of diabetes, a history of previous macrosomic babies, history of previous gestational diabetes, previous unexplained stillbirth, polyhydramnios or macrosomia or maternal obesity. While some units perform routine screening in all pregnant women using a random blood sugar, others select only those women with clinical risk factors (Table 7.2).

An oral glucose test (75-g glucose) can be employed to confirm the diagnosis, although the world-wide diversity of criteria for the diagnosis of gestational diabetes is problematic (SIGN 1996; Meltzer *et al.* 1998). Gestational diabetes can be diagnosed with a 75-g glucose load when two of the following three values are met or exceeded.

- fasting glucose > 5.3 mmol/l
- one-hour glucose level > 10.6 mmol/l
- two-hour glucose level > 8.9 mmol/l.

Table 7.2 Indications for glucose tolerance test

- Glycosuria × 2 on fasting specimens
- Strong family history of diabetes
- Previous macrosomic baby
- Previous gestational diabetes
- Previous unexplained stillbirth
- Polyhydramnios
- Maternal obesity
- Macrosomic fetus/large for dates

Impaired glucose tolerance of pregnancy is diagnosed if only one value is met or exceeded (Table 7.3).

The importance of gestational diabetes is that:

- women with the condition may have an increased incidence of adverse pregnancy outcomes
- it identifies a cohort of women who have a highly significant risk (40–60%) of developing NIDDM in the future
- some women with an abnormal glucose tolerance test will have undiagnosed IDDM.

There is a small increase in perinatal mortality in gestational diabetes. This may not be caused by the gestational diabetes but instead may be independently related to maternal obesity, a large fetus or previous poor obstetric outcome that may have prompted the glucose tolerance test.

Table 7.3 75-g oral glucose-tolerance test results in pregnancy (data from Meltzer et al. 1998)

	Value		
	Fasting (> 5.3 mmol/l)	One-hour (> 10.6 mmol/l)	Two-hour (> 8.9 mmol/l)
Gestational diabetes	Diagnosis is made when two of the three values are met or exceeded		
Impaired glucose intolerance	Diagnosis is made when one of the three values is met or exceeded		

Despite the controversy surrounding the diagnosis of gestational diabetes and 'impaired glucose tolerance', most units in the UK treat the condition. There is, however, no clear evidence that treatment reduces perinatal morbidity or mortality. When insulin plus dietary modifications were compared with dietary modifications alone, there was a decrease in macrosomia in the former group, but no effect on caesarean section rates, shoulder dystocia or perinatal mortality (Langer *et al.* 1989).

Women identified as having impaired glucose tolerance or gestational diabetes should attend specialist clinics managed by both obstetricians and physicians. Dietary advice will be the mainstay of treatment for most of these women, although some women with persistent hyperglycaemia will require insulin. Careful blood glucose monitoring should occur as in pregnancies complicated by IDDM. Women with gestational diabetes are at increased risk of pre-eclampsia and their blood pressure and urinalysis should be checked regularly. Assessment of fetal growth and well-being should be performed at least at fortnightly intervals in the third trimester and may influence the mode of delivery if macrosomia is identified. It is, however, of interest that the diagnosis of gestational diabetes increases a woman's chance of delivery by caesarean section with no proven benefit for the neonate.

Postnatally, these women should have a formal glucose tolerance test performed to assess whether they are diabetic or have a degree of glucose intolerance outwith pregnancy. Further, they should be counselled about their risks of developing diabetes in the future, made aware of the symptoms of diabetes and advised of the benefits of losing weight and altering their lifestyles accordingly. Their risk of developing gestational diabetes in a future pregnancy is significant.

Thyroid disease

PHYSIOLOGY

During pregnancy, increased circulating oestrogen levels stimulate the hepatic production of thyroid-binding globulin (TBG). TBG levels reach their peak by 24 weeks of gestation and remain elevated until two weeks after delivery. To compensate for this rise in TBG, total levels of circulating tri-iodothyronine (T_3) and thyroxine (T_4) are increased. An evaluation of thyroid function during pregnancy therefore requires an assessment of free T_3 and free T_4. Both free T_3 and free T_4 are slightly elevated in the first trimester and thyroid-stimulating hormone (TSH) is decreased; in 10–15% of normal women, TSH is suppressed into the hyperthyroid range. This may, in part, be due to the production of human chorionic gonadotrophin (hCG) by the placenta, which is structurally similar to TSH and does have some thyrotrophic activity. In the third trimester of pregnancy, concentrations of free T_3 and free T_4 are reduced and TSH concentration is increased. This may be due to a decline in thyroid stimulation by hCG in later pregnancy or to the relative iodine deficiency that exists then. This relative iodine deficiency arises because of both an increased urinary excretion and increased demands of the fetus. A goitre may develop to trap sufficient iodine in women with a dietary insufficiency.

HYPERTHYROIDISM

Hyperthyroidism is a relatively common medical condition, which occurs in around 1:500 pregnancies. Most are secondary to Grave's disease (95%), an autoimmune disorder where the thyroid is stimulated by antibodies directed against the TSH receptor. The clinical features of hyperthyroidism, which include weight loss, palpitations, tremor, increased appetite, vomiting, goitre, heat intolerance and altered bowel function, are common in normal pregnancy. The diagnosis of hyperthyroidism is made biochemically, by detecting a raised free T_3 or free T_4. TSH levels will be suppressed, although this can occur in normal pregnancy.

Effect of pregnancy on hyperthyroidism

Like most autoimmune conditions, Grave's disease often improves during pregnancy, although the increased thyroid activity that occurs in the first trimester can worsen the disease. An exacerbation can also occur postpartum and is associated with increasing levels of TSH receptor-stimulating antibodies.

Effect of hyperthyroidism on pregnancy

Well-controlled patients rarely have problems during pregnancy. Severe, uncontrolled disease is associated with anovulatory infertility. Those thyrotoxic women who manage to conceive have an increased risk of pregnancy complications (Table 7.4). Serial ultrasound scans should be performed in the third trimester to assess fetal growth. Other fetal problems relate to the transfer of thyroid-stimulating antibodies from mother to fetus, which can provoke fetal hyperthyroidism. This rarely causes significant problems especially if the mother is on antithyroid medication, as this will suppress fetal thyroid activity, but neonatal thyrotoxicosis can occur in around 10% of babies of mothers with Grave's disease.

The major risk to the mother is congestive cardiac failure and a thyroid crisis. These complications can be precipitated by infection or stress and

Table 7.4 Pregnancy complications associated with thyrotoxicosis

- Spontaneous miscarriage
- Chromosomal abnormalities
- Intrauterine growth restriction
- Preterm delivery
- Increased perinatal mortality

are characterised by tachycardia and hyperpyrexia, vomiting, diarrhoea and central nervous system dysfunction. Rarely, a goitre can enlarge during pregnancy to cause a degree of tracheal obstruction that may be detected only during intubation.

MANAGEMENT OF HYPERTHYROIDISM

The aim of treatment during pregnancy is to render the woman euthyroid to control maternal symptoms, avoid serious maternal complications, such as cardiac failure, and to protect the fetus from the complications listed above. Radioactive iodine therapy is contraindicated during pregnancy and for mothers who are breastfeeding, since the radio-iodine is sequestered by the fetal thyroid gland, resulting in ablation and hypothyroidism. Pregnancy should not be contemplated for at least four months after radio-iodine treatment.

Antithyroid drugs, and in particular the thioureas, are the mainstay of treatment for hyperthyroidism during pregnancy. Carbimazole and propylthiouracil are the drugs most commonly used in the UK and methimazole, a metabolite of carbimazole, is the drug most commonly employed in the USA. After the diagnosis of Grave's disease is made, most courses of antithyroid drugs are given for 12–18 months, although up to 50% of patients relapse and require long-term treatment. Thiourea drugs act by inhibiting the organification of iodine and the coupling of iodothyronines in the thyroid. Both drugs readily cross the placenta and, although neither is teratogenic, carbimazole has been associated with a rare scalp defect, aplasia cutis. Carbimazole and propylthiouracil will affect the fetal thyroid and, in high doses, these drugs may cause fetal hypothyroidism and goitre. Maternal adverse effects of the thioureas include skin rash (1%), arthralgia and gastrointestinal symptoms. The most serious adverse effect is granulocytopenia, usually dose-related and occurring within two months of commencing treatment. Women should be advised to report a skin rash or sore throat immediately.

Antithyroid drugs can be continued during breastfeeding. Carbimazole and methimazole are excreted in breast milk in significant amounts but do not seem to alter neonatal thyroid function in low doses (less than 30 mg/day). Since less propylthiouracil crosses the placenta and is excreted in breast milk, this drug is probably preferable for newly diagnosed cases of hyperthyroidism in pregnancy.

Beta-blockers are commonly employed in the initial management of thyrotoxicosis to control tachycardia and tremor. These agents should be discontinued when the woman is euthyroid since long-term administration is associated with intrauterine growth restriction. Where patients do not respond to drug therapy or there is a serious intolerance along with significant disease, partial thyroidectomy may be required. Surgery is also indicated in the rare situations where thyroid carcinoma is diagnosed or where an enlarging goitre is compressing surrounding structures. It is usual to pretreat patients with iodine therapy for seven to ten days to decrease the vascularity of the gland and prevent a thyroid crisis. The use of a beta-blocker may also help control the symptoms preoperatively.

HYPOTHYROIDISM

Hypothyroidism complicates about 1% of pregnancies and most women will have had the diagnosis made and be on appropriate treatment prior to conception. Severe hypothyroidism tends to result in oligo- or amenorrhoea with a high incidence of anovulatory infertility. Most women who conceive are therefore on thyroxine supplements. The most common causes of hypothyroidism in young women are Hashimoto's thyroiditis and atrophic thyroiditis, which are associated with the presence of circulating autoantibodies. The symptoms of hypothyroidism include tiredness, weight gain, constipation, fluid retention, hair loss, dry skin and carpal tunnel syndrome and again these are commonly found in normal pregnancy. The diagnosis is confirmed biochemically by identifying a low free T_4 and a raised TSH. Thyroid function tests should be monitored at least once per trimester to ensure adequate replacement of thyroxine.

Effect of pregnancy on hypothyroidism

Pregnancy has little or no effect on hypothyroidism and, in most women, the dose of thyroxine replacement will remain unchanged. The need for an increased dose of T_4 may, in part, be related to whether the hypothyroidism is due to ablation by radio-iodine or surgery for previous thyrotoxicosis or to primary autoimmune hypothyroidism. The former is more likely to require an increase in dose. Some clinicians increase thyroxine dosage in early pregnancy in line with the normal physiological increase in free T_3 and free T_4 to ensure an adequate supply of thyroid hormone to the fetus. Others advocate an increase in the late second and third trimesters to take account of the weight gain during pregnancy. Should dose adjustment occur during pregnancy, this should be reassessed following delivery. Usual management at the Glasgow Royal Infirmary is to check thyroid function tests at booking and correct any under- or over-replacement. Thyroid function tests are then monitored at least in each trimester with dose adjustment if TSH is elevated and free T_4 low. More frequent monitoring is required following dose adjustment.

Effect of hypothyroidism on pregnancy

It is unusual for hypothyroidism to cause significant problems in pregnancy. Severe and uncontrolled disease is associated with an increased risk of spontaneous miscarriage, perinatal mortality, pre-eclampsia and intrauterine growth restriction. Some studies have found an increased incidence of congenital abnormalities in uncontrolled hypothyroidism. Hypothyroidism in pregnancy may result in subsequent developmental problems in the child. For the majority of women on adequate replacement, hypothyroidism is associated with a normal maternal and fetal outcome.

PROLACTINOMA

Pregnancy is normally associated with a substantial increase in circulating prolactin levels of around ten-fold. It is likely that this reflects hyperplasia of the pituitary lactotrophs due to the high oestrogen levels associated with pregnancy. There is also an increase in volume of the pituitary gland (up to 35%) during pregnancy. These elevated levels of prolactin return to normal when breastfeeding is discontinued.

Effect of pregnancy on prolactinoma

Prolactinomas are the most commonly encountered pituitary tumours in pregnancy. They can be either microprolactinomas (less than 1 cm) or macroprolactinomas ($\geqslant 1$ cm). Since the pituitary gland enlarges during pregnancy, there is a small risk that the oestrogenic stimulation will provoke tumour expansion, leading to headache, visual field defects or the development of diabetes insipidus. It is unusual for patients with microadenomas to have a clinically significant expansion in their tumour during pregnancy (risk less than 2%), although the risk for macroadenomas is much greater (15%). This latter figure can be reduced (to less than 5%) if the tumour has been treated prior to conception, and reduction in tumour size should be confirmed objectively by pituitary imaging prior to pregnancy.

Effect of prolactinoma on pregnancy

Women with hyperprolactinaemia due to prolactinoma will clearly have a problem with fertility, although ovulation is likely to return to normal following treatment with the dopamine receptor agonists, bromocriptine or cabergoline. When these patients become pregnant these treatments should be discontinued. The patient should be made aware of the risk of tumour expansion and the need to report severe headache or change in vision during the pregnancy. Monitoring of prolactin levels during pregnancy can be difficult to interpret owing to the 10- to 20-fold increase in prolactin levels during the course of normal pregnancy. There is a place for regular assessment of visual fields, although this is unlikely to show any abnormality in the asymptomatic patient. Should symptoms occur, tumour size and expansion should be determined by CT or magnetic resonance imaging; dopamine-receptor agonists can be reintroduced with no adverse effects on the pregnancy. Breastfeeding is not contraindicated in patients with prolactinomas or in women on dopamine-receptor agonists, although these agents may inhibit milk production.

References

Langer, O., Anyaegbunam, A., Brustman, L. and Divon, M. (1989) Management of women with one abnormal glucose tolerance test value reduces adverse outcome in pregnancy. *Am J Obstet Gynecol* **161**, 593–9

Meltzer, S., Leiter, L., Daneman, D. *et al.* (1998) 1998 clinical practice guidelines for the management of diabetes in Canada. *CMAJ* **159** suppl 8, 51–29

SIGN (Scottish Intercollegiate Guidelines Network) (1996) *Management of Diabetes in Pregnancy.* Edinburgh: SIGN (SIGN Publication no. 9)

(II) HEART DISEASE

Changes in the cardiovascular system in normal pregnancy

There is an increase in plasma volume with a lesser rise in red cell volume leading to the physiological anaemia of pregnancy. Total blood volume may increase by up to 50% during pregnancy with an increase starting in the early part of the first trimester. Cardiac output also increases by up to 50% again starting from early in pregnancy. The increase in cardiac output is mainly brought about by an increase in stroke volume with a small increase in resting heart rate. These changes are accompanied by a fall in peripheral resistance so explaining the reduction in blood pressure that occurs in the course of normal pregnancy.

Blood pressure falls to reach a nadir at 20 weeks of gestation, then gradually climbs again, to levels compatible with the nonpregnant situation, by the mid to late part of the third trimester. In the third trimester, the gravid uterus may inhibit venous return, particularly in supine positions, thus compromising cardiac output. Turning from the lateral to the supine position may result in a 25% reduction in cardiac output. On examination, the pregnant woman may be noted to have warm extremities with dilated veins and, on auscultation, it is not uncommon for a third heart sound and an ejection systolic flow murmur to be heard, due to the hyperdynamic circulation of pregnancy.

EFFECT OF HEART DISEASE ON PREGNANCY

Heart disease can have important effects on pregnancy. Medications employed in the management of heart disease can affect the fetus. Beta-blockers are associated with intrauterine growth restriction, while the anticoagulant warfarin is teratogenic and can have adverse effects on the fetus throughout pregnancy (see also Section XIII Table 7.23). The fetus of the cardiac patient is at risk of intrauterine growth restriction and preterm delivery, which may be associated with maternal hypoxia. Women with more severe heart disease (New York Heart Association class III or IV; Table 7.5) are more likely to have a poor pregnancy outcome. When the woman's heart disease is congenital, her fetus is at increased risk of having a congenital heart defect. This risk is about

Table 7.5 New York Heart Association Classification of heart disease	
Grade	Symptoms
I	Patients with cardiac disease but no cardiac decompensation. There is no limitation during ordinary physical exercise
II	No symptoms of cardiac decompensation at rest but slight limitation by dyspnoea with activities such as walking
III	Marked limitation of physical activity although no cardiac symptoms at rest
IV	Breathlessness at rest

5–10% and depends upon the specific lesion. Marfan syndrome has an autosomal dominant inheritance.

EFFECT OF PREGNANCY ON HEART DISEASE

Normal physiological changes in the cardiovascular system in pregnancy (increased cardiac output and increased stroke volume) may aggravate underlying cardiac disease. There are certain conditions, including complicated coarctation of the aorta, Eisenmenger's syndrome and Marfan syndrome with aortic involvement, which are associated with significant maternal mortality. Pregnancy has a particularly serious effect on women with fixed pulmonary vascular resistance who are unable to increase pulmonary blood flow to match the increased cardiac output.

Presentation of heart disease in pregnancy

In modern practice rheumatic heart disease is rapidly declining and the number of patients with congenital heart disease is increasing. Most women will know at the time of presentation in pregnancy of their history of heart disease and this should be evident on history taking. It is unusual to identify a previously undiagnosed major cardiac problem in pregnancy. However, as rheumatic heart disease remains common in other countries, immigrant women with undiagnosed heart disease may present for the first time in pregnancy. A history of dyspnoea, both on exertion and at rest, and syncope should be sought and, on examination, care should be taken to identify any scars from previous cardiac surgery and any thrills or murmurs.

Important factors to assess both in the prepregnancy counselling of women with heart disease and in the assessment of women with heart disease during pregnancy are the severity of heart disease by the New York Heart Association Classification (Table 7.5) and the presence of pulmonary hypertension and cyanosis. Regardless of its aetiology, patients who are asymptomatic prior to pregnancy and have only grade I or II levels of symptoms on the New York Heart Association Classification are unlikely to have major problems during a pregnancy. Particular concern should be given to women with pulmonary hypertension, mitral stenosis and Marfan syndrome. Pulmonary hypertension secondary to Eisenmenger's syndrome has an associated maternal mortality of 30–50%.

Valvular heart disease

Many patients with valvular heart disease will have had a valve replacement prior to pregnancy. This is usually a mechanical valve, as bioprosthetic valves deteriorate more rapidly and are not usually used in young women. The main consideration with valvular heart disease, where mechanical valves are in place, is that of anticoagulation. Warfarin places the patient at increased risk of warfarin embryopathy. This appears, in part, to be related to dose, and fetal bleeding, particularly at the time of delivery (see also Section xiii Table 7.23). However, transferring to heparin can be troublesome and may be associated with an increased risk of valve thrombosis. In order to avoid the risk of warfarin embryopathy, transfer to heparin would have to occur by six weeks. Often, this is impractical unless prepregnancy counselling has established both the need to do this and a management plan. Where warfarin is continued, the patient should be aware of the risk of warfarin embryopathy, which is estimated at around 6.4% but may be lower with smaller doses of warfarin and good control. Thus, it is better for the patient to undergo prepregnancy counselling prior to facing these problems in pregnancy.

The risk of fetal bleeding with warfarin also has to be appreciated. This is particularly high at the time of delivery and usually these patients will be admitted in the late third trimester and switched to therapeutic doses of heparin in anticipation of delivery, which may be organised electively. Some women prefer to avoid any risk to the baby and wish to stay on heparin throughout pregnancy. This is provided by twice daily therapeutic doses of heparin subcutaneously with a mid-interval activated partial prothrombin time of 2.0 (1.5–2.5). There have been reports of low molecular weight heparin, in therapeutic doses, being used in such patients without any thrombotic problem. However, there is insufficient information at present to routinely advocate this and it should, at least at present, be restricted to specialist centres. The patient must also be aware that she would be at risk of the adverse effects of heparin, particularly heparin-induced osteoporosis (see also Section xiii Table 7.23).

Occasionally, mitral stenosis is encountered in pregnancy. The main risk is of pulmonary oedema developing, which may be triggered by problems such as chest infection and situations where tachycardia occurs. This arises because there is less time to allow adequate left ventricular filling and a subsequent backing-up of blood in the left atrium and lungs. Reduction in the heart rate by use of beta-blockers will increase the left ventricle filling time with subsequent increases in stroke volume. Should there be a significant deterioration then surgical treatment may be required by techniques such as balloon valvotomy or closed mitral valvotomy

Situations where the patient has to be placed on cardiopulmonary bypass, such as during the valve replacement, place the fetus at considerable risk and ideally should not be performed during pregnancy. The treatment of pulmonary oedema where it arises is similar to that in the nonpregnant situation and diuretics should be administered. If atrial fibrillation occurs then digoxin can be given and consideration should be given to anticoagulation to prevent development of atrial thrombus.

Congenital heart disease

The most common forms of congenital heart disease encountered during pregnancy are atrial septal defect, ventricular septal defect and patent ductus arteriosus, which account for about two-thirds of cases. Patients with acyanotic congenital heart disease generally do well in pregnancy (Table 7.6).

Table 7.6 Congenital heart disease in pregnancy	
Defect	*Toleration in pregnancy*
Atrial septal defect	Usually well tolerated in pregnancy
Ventricular septal defect	Well tolerated unless complicated by Eisenmenger's syndrome
Patent ductus arteriosus	Most cases will have undergone surgical correction
	Uncorrected cases with no pulmonary hypertension usually do well
Congenital aortic stenosis	May be problematic if gradient is greater than 100 mmHg
	Balloon valvotomy can be employed during pregnancy
Marfan syndrome	Major complications include: aortic dilatation, aortic rupture, and increasing mitral or aortic regurgitation
	Beta-blockers can reduce the risk of complications
Coarctation of the aorta	Usually corrected before pregnancy
	Uncorrected coarctation associated with aortic rupture, aortic dissection, angina, hypertension and heart failure

Often, the congenital heart disease will have been corrected. Fallot's tetralogy, a form of cyanotic congenital heart disease, is generally well tolerated in pregnancy. Concerns include the effects of maternal hypoxia (which may worsen during pregnancy) on the fetus, which include intrauterine growth restriction, preterm delivery and spontaneous miscarriage, and paradoxical emboli. Thromboprophylaxis should be employed to reduce the risk of the latter. Significant problems tend to occur where there is pulmonary hypertension, which may be primary or due to the development of Eisenmenger's syndrome. These women should be offered termination of pregnancy and, if they decline this, they require intensive antenatal care by a combined obstetric, cardiology and anaesthetic service. Even with optimal care, Eisenmenger's syndrome carries a significant risk of maternal mortality (50%).

Cardiomyopathy

The most common cardiomyopathy seen is hypertrophic cardiomyopathy. These patients often cope reasonably well with pregnancy and are usually treated with beta-blocking drugs to allow adequate time for ventricular filling. As a consequence of this treatment, these women will be at risk of intrauterine fetal growth restriction. Similarly, epidural anaesthesia is usually avoided as it reduces the afterload, so in turn reducing left ventricular filling. Puerperal cardiomyopathy is a rare complication of pregnancy, usually occurring four to six weeks postnatally. It is characterised by palpitation, dyspnoea, oedema (peripheral and central) and an impaired exercise tolerance; the diagnosis is confirmed on echocardiography. The management includes treatment of heart failure, anticoagulation and, in selected cases, immunosuppressive therapy. However, some women fail to respond to these measures and heart transplantation should be considered.

(III) SKIN DISORDERS

Physiology

Normal changes occur within the skin in pregnancy. Spider naevi, palmar erythema and striae gravidarum are commonplace and a mild degree of gum hypertrophy and gingivitis may occur. Beginning in the first trimester, increased pigmentation can occur on the face (chloasma), on the areolae and axillae and as a prominent linea nigra on the abdomen. Hair growth can increase, although alopecia can occur and is a common feature postnatally. Normal pregnancy may be associated with pruritis in the absence of a rash or abnormal liver function tests. Liver function tests should always be performed in pregnant women with pruritus to exclude intrahepatic cholestasis of pregnancy (see Section IX).

Polymorphic eruption of pregnancy

Also known as pruritic urticarial papules and plaques of pregnancy (PUPPP), this condition occurs in about one in 250 pregnancies late in the third trimester. It presents as intensely itchy papules and plaques on the abdomen, upper limbs and buttocks. It resolves rapidly postnatally and has no adverse effects on the fetus. Treatment includes topical steroids, oral antihistamines and, occasionally, oral steroids. Topical preparations of menthol in aqueous cream or phenol in calamine may provide symptomatic relief.

Prurigo of pregnancy

This is an itchy papular eruption that occurs in around one in 300 pregnancies. It is not associated with any adverse risks to the mother or the fetus. It usually begins in the early part of the third trimester and is manifest as discrete itchy papules over the extensor surfaces of the limbs and the abdomen. It is not vesicular in nature. Oral antihistamines and topical steroid creams are of value in controlling it.

Pemphigoid gestationis

Pemphigoid gestationis, previously named herpes gestationis, is a more worrying condition in pregnancy. This is a rare condition (1: 10 000 to 1: 60 000 pregnancies) which may be associated with autoimmune disease. It usually starts in the second trimester with itching preceding a widespread polymorphic eruption with vesicles and bullae formation. Pruritus is a major symptom and definitive diagnosis can be made with skin biopsy demonstrating complement deposition at the basement membrane. This condition is associated with intrauterine growth restriction and preterm delivery. Treatment includes oral antihistamines to relieve the itch, topical steroids and, if severe, oral steroids will be required. Since oral corticosteroid treatment is itself associated with intrauterine growth restriction, serial ultrasound scans should be performed to assess fetal growth. This condition has a tendency to recur in future pregnancies and sometimes with oral contraceptive use.

Pruritic folliculitis

This condition presents as a widespread pruritic eruption predominantly on the trunk and thighs. The eruption is acneiform in nature, with follicular papules and pustules. It usually presents in the latter half of pregnancy and resolves in the early puerperium. Pruritic folliculitis is not associated with any adverse effects on the fetus. Treatment is with topical benzoyl peroxide, antihistamines and, occasionally, topical steroids.

(IV) INFECTION

Urinary tract infection

Urinary tract infection (acute cystitis and pyelonephritis) is one of the most common medical complications of pregnancy, occurring in about 1–2% of pregnancies. The organism most commonly identified in urinary tract infection during pregnancy is *Escherichia coli* (in up to 90% and often ampicillin-resistant) ascending from the perineum. Between 2% and 10% of women have significant numbers of bacteria (more than 100 000 organisms per ml) in their urine during pregnancy, usually without exhibiting any symptoms (asymptomatic bacteriuria). This is a potentially serious complication since 15–45% of these women, if left untreated, will develop pyelonephritis, which is associated with an increase in maternal and fetal morbidity. Screening and treating all pregnant women for asymptomatic bacteriuria is effective and cost-beneficial in reducing the risk of pyelonephritis. Further, it appears to reduce the risk of preterm delivery and low birth weight, although the mechanism whereby treatment of bacteriuria does this remains uncertain. The antibiotic used to treat asymptomatic bacteriuria will depend on the sensitivities of the causative organism. Most clinicians continue antimicrobial treatment for between one and two weeks, although at present there is insufficient evidence to give guidance on the optimum duration of treatment.

Acute cystitis is characterised by urinary frequency, dysuria and lower abdominal pain. Haematuria and proteinuria are identified on urinalysis. The diagnosis is confirmed by finding significant bacteriuria on culture of a midstream specimen of urine. Acute cystitis should be treated with a course of antibiotics, simple analgesics and an increased fluid intake. Regular follow-up urine cultures should be obtained after completing antimicrobial therapy to exclude reinfection. Recurrent urinary tract infection during pregnancy usually merits antibiotic prophylaxis with an appropriate antibiotic taken at night to allow it maximum time in the bladder. As recurrent urinary tract infection may be secondary to an underlying abnormality of the urinary tract, radiological assessment should be considered postnatally.

Acute pyelonephritis is more common during pregnancy because of the physiological dilatation of the upper renal tract. It is suspected clinically by the presence of dysuria, loin pain, lower abdominal pain, fever and rigors, and is confirmed by a positive urine culture. Blood should be obtained for a full blood count and for culture before treatment is commenced. The management of this condition includes hospitalisation, intravenous fluids and analgesia. Intravenous antibiotics are commenced before the results of urine culture and, since the infection is most probably due to *E. coli*, a cephalosporin is the initial choice. Combination therapy with a cephalosporin and an aminoglycoside is appropriate in women who are seriously unwell or when there are concerns about antibiotic resistance. Careful monitoring of aminoglycoside levels is required during pregnancy to avoid fetal ototoxicity. An ultrasound examination of the woman's kidneys is required to exclude an underlying renal disorder, which can predispose to pyelonephritis. It must be noted however that a marked degree of dilatation of the ureters occurs in pregnancy, particularly on the right.

Rubella

Rubella is a mildly infectious disease, previously common among children aged four to nine years. It is characterised by a transient erythematous rash, lymphadenopathy involving post-auricular and sub-occipital glands and, occasionally in adults, arthritis and arthralgia. The incubation period is 14–21 days and the period of infectivity is from one week before until four days after the onset of rash. Rubella was made a notifiable disease in the UK in 1988. Clinical diagnosis is unreliable and the rash is not diagnostic of rubella. Therefore, confirmation of acute rubella infection is recommended in all suspected cases and, while saliva samples may be appropriate for men, nonpregnant women and children, serological samples are essential for pregnant women.

Maternal rubella infection in the first trimester of pregnancy is associated with adverse fetal effects in up to 90% of infants. The risk of fetal damage declines to about 10–20% by 16 weeks of gestation and is extremely rare thereafter. Fetal defects associated with maternal rubella infection are listed in Table 7.7. Termination of pregnancy should be offered when maternal infection is confirmed in the first 16 weeks of pregnancy.

The objective of rubella immunisation programmes is to prevent infection during pregnancy and congenital rubella syndrome (CRS). Before the introduction of rubella immunisation, there were up to 70 cases of CRS during epidemic years with perhaps a further 700 therapeutic terminations. Two approaches to rubella immunisation have been used in the UK: selective immunisation of pre-pubertal girls and nonimmune women and universal immunisation of young children. The former policy, introduced in 1970, increased the proportion of women with anti-

Table 7.7 Fetal effects of maternal first-trimester rubella infection
• Fetal death
• Intrauterine growth restriction
• Deafness
• Cataract, glaucoma, microphthalmia
• Jaundice
• Thrombocytopenic purpura
• Hepatosplenomegaly
• Mental handicap
• Congenital heart disease
• Inflammatory lesions of lung, brain, liver and bone-marrow

bodies to rubella from 85–90% to 97–98%. However, the few remaining rubella-susceptible women continued to be exposed to rubella by their own and friends' children. Since 1988, it has been recommended that all boys and girls should be immunised with rubella-containing vaccine (MMR) at 12–15 months of age and again at approximately four years. As a result, the number of CRS cases has fallen to around five annually.

All pregnant women with suspected rubella or exposure to rubella should be investigated serologically. A blood sample should be taken as soon as possible after the exposure to rubella and sent to the laboratory with a detailed history of the last menstrual period and date of exposure. Close collaboration between virologist and obstetrician is necessary to interpret the serological results accurately. In summary, if a blood specimen is taken from the woman less than ten days from exposure to rubella, her rubella-specific IgG level will be determined in order to assess her susceptibility. If blood is taken after ten days from exposure an increase in rubella-specific IgM, which does not usually persist for more than two months, indicates active or recent infection.

Pregnant women who are found not to be immune early in pregnancy should be immunised postnatally during a period of contraception. Pregnant women should not be given the rubella vaccine, although available data indicate that the risk of teratogenicity from the live vaccine is virtually non-existent.

Syphilis

Infectious syphilis during pregnancy is particularly important as it usually results in miscarriage, stillbirth or in a congenitally infected baby. Congenital infection is associated with long-term morbidity including learning difficulties, interstitial keratitis and neural deafness. Risk of vertical transmission diminishes as maternal syphilis advances, but in the early latent (asymptomatic) stages, the risk of transmission remains about 30–60%. In the UK, antenatal serological screening for syphilis is routinely performed. This allows detection of maternal infection, treatment with penicillin and the prevention of vertical transmission. Although syphilis is uncommon in this country, a programme of screening and treating is cost-effective: 139 women were diagnosed with and treated for syphilis in pregnancy between 1994 and 1997. Treatment of mothers should consist of antibiotics, preferably a penicillin. The woman's sexual partner and infant should be followed up and treated, if infected.

Chickenpox (varicella zoster)

Infection with the varicella zoster virus and the development of chickenpox is common in childhood. Only about 2% of reported cases of chickenpox occur in people over the age of 20 years, although the infection tends to be more severe in these people. While chickenpox is uncommon in pregnancy, (1/2000 pregnancies), contact with an infected person is not infrequent and causes anxiety and concern for the pregnant woman. Some studies have suggested that infection during pregnancy is more severe than in nonpregnant controls, although this may reflect a reporting bias. Certainly there is an association with maternal pneumonitis and subsequent calcification in the lungs.

Severe varicella infection can result in fetal death and preterm labour, which are both non-specific effects related to the severity of the maternal illness. Overall, there is no increase in the incidence of congenital abnormality following maternal varicella infection. However, varicella can cross the placenta and infect the fetus. This can, albeit rarely, result in a characteristic syndrome (Table 7.8). Prospective studies have indicated that the risk of the fetal varicella syndrome after maternal chickenpox in the first trimester is about 3%.

Maternal varicella infection late in pregnancy is associated with neonatal infection in up to 60% of cases. This is usually mild and a rash may be present at birth or develop in the first few days of life. However, when the onset of maternal infection occurs between five days before and two days after delivery, the neonatal infection may be more severe, with mortality rates of 30% reported. The severity of infection may be due to fetal infection without the protection of maternal antibodies.

Table 7.8 Features of fetal varicella syndrome
• Limb hypoplasia
• Cicatricial limb lesions with a dermatomal distribution
• Neurological abnormalities (hydrocephalus and microcephaly)
• Eye abnormalities (Horner syndrome, cataracts, chorioretinitis, microphthalmia)
• Gastrointestinal and genitourinary defects
• Intrauterine growth restriction

Pregnant women who are exposed to varicella should have their susceptibility confirmed using an assay of serum antibodies. If they have not had a previous infection, they should be given zoster immunoglobulin, which can modify or prevent clinical infection. There is no evidence that it can prevent fetal infection or damage. If exposure occurs in pregnancy, an ultrasound scan should be performed to assess fetal anatomy. Zoster immunoglobulin should also be given to neonates whose mothers develop chickenpox within a few days of delivery. Severe or progressive maternal or neonatal varicella infection should be treated with intravenous acyclovir.

Parvovirus B19

Parvovirus B19 is typically a mild, febrile childhood infection that follows a benign course (erythema infectiosum or slapped-cheek syndrome). Symptomless infection is common and about 30–40% of the population have antibodies to the virus. In adults, the infection is less common and tends to be more severe with a high incidence of arthralgia. In 1984, parvovirus B19 was identified as a fetal pathogen when the first case of hydrops fetalis associated with maternal infection was reported. The virus can replicate in bone marrow cells to inhibit erythropoiesis. The risk of acquiring parvovirus B19 during pregnancy, averaged over epidemic and non-epidemic years, is about 1/400. Infection during the first 20 weeks of pregnancy is associated with an increased risk of fetal loss (spontaneous miscarriage and intrauterine death) of 9%. The risk of those infected during weeks 9–20 of gestation developing fetal hydrops is 3%. The virus is not associated with fetal developmental abnormalities or any long-term effects on the child's health.

During epidemics, pregnant women should be educated about the infection and advised to avoid exposure where possible. Women who work in close contact with children are at particular risk of infection.

Human immunodeficiency virus

Human immunodeficiency virus (HIV) is a relatively new, fatal, sexually transmitted disease which is likely to have infected 40 million people, mostly in the third world, by the year 2000. One quarter of these will be children, the majority of whom will have acquired their infection as a result of mother-to-child transmission. The virus is most prevalent in East and Central Africa where, in some areas, up to 30% of pregnant women are infected. Prevalence rates remain low in the UK, although anonymous testing during pregnancy has shown rates of 0.5% in inner London.

Pregnancy does not seem to have a major adverse effect on HIV progression and the survival time of women with acquired immune deficiency syndrome (AIDS) is not affected by pregnancy. Infection may increase the rate of early pregnancy loss, perhaps by altering the population of immune cells within the decidua. The rate of fetal abnormality does not appear to be influenced by the virus. Studies from developing countries have indicated that HIV infection is associated with intrauterine growth restriction, preterm delivery and an increase in perinatal mortality. Infectious complications are more common in women with advanced HIV disease.

Rates of vertical transmission of the virus to the fetus vary from 15–20% in Europe, 15–30% in the USA and 25–35% in Africa. Rates of transmission may be related to viral load, although other factors including maternal immunological status, advanced clinical disease and prolonged rupture of the fetal membranes, seem to be involved. Transmission can occur during pregnancy, during delivery or postnatally during breastfeeding. Most vertical transmission (60–70%) occurs during delivery, although breastfeeding can add another 7–22% risk of transmission. Interventions aimed at reducing the rates of vertical transmission are a priority if childhood mortality from the HIV virus is to be reduced and numerous strategies have been proposed (Table 7.9).

Zidovudine (previously azidothymidine, AZT) monotherapy has been shown to reduce the risk of vertical transmission from 26% to 8% in asymptomatic French and American women with relatively high counts of the T lymphocyte population CD4. In this trial, oral zidovudine was given to women antenatally and intravenously during labour and their infants were given oral treatment postnatally. There are concerns, however, that monotherapy zidovudine might not be in the best inter-

Table 7.9 Strategies to reduce vertical transmission of HIV in pregnancy

- Antiretroviral therapy (single agent or combination therapy)[a]
- Delivery by caesarean section[a]
- Avoidance of breastfeeding[a]
- Vaginal lavage
- Delayed artificial rupture of the fetal membranes
- Avoidance of episiotomy, instrumental delivery and fetal scalp electrodes
- Immunotherapy with hyperimmune globulin
- Vitamin A supplementation[a]

[a] shown to have a proven benefit

ests of the mother since it may lead to viral mutation with the emergence of zidovudine-resistant viral strains. Further studies are required to confirm that zidovudine has no adverse effects on the fetus. Also, the drug is expensive and will not be affordable by those countries with the highest transmission rates. Recent studies have demonstrated that delivery by caesarean section in women infected with HIV cuts rates of vertical transmission by up to 50%.

Breastfeeding should be discouraged in HIV-positive women in developed countries although, in developing countries, breastfeeding may be a safer option than formula feeding for these women.

ANTENATAL SCREENING FOR HIV

Even though the prevalence of HIV in the UK remains relatively low and has certainly not reached predicted proportions, a significant number of women infected with HIV remain undetected. Anonymous antenatal screening in London and the South-East indicates that 87% of HIV positive women are unaware of their status. Testing for HIV infection in hospital and community antenatal clinics has been unsuccessful, despite Department of Health guidelines. Since interventions are now available which can decrease the risk of vertical transmission, a policy of universal HIV screening in early pregnancy now seems appropriate. Furthermore, antenatal identification of women who are HIV positive would allow the early identification of infected infants, thereby optimising their management. Approximately 300 babies are born with HIV infection in the UK each year and the majority of them are diagnosed late. In the absence of a universal screening programme, women at high-risk should be offered screening.

Toxoplasmosis

Toxoplasma gondii is a protozoal parasite that infects cats as the definitive host and mice as the intermediate host. Other animals, including sheep, cattle and pigs can serve as intermediate hosts. Women can acquire the parasite by contact with cats, ingestion of foods contaminated with oocytes or undercooked meat. Maternal infection during pregnancy may result in congenital infection in the infant, sometimes with serious sequelae. In most cases, maternal infection is asymptomatic, but acute infection may be associated with fever, cough, malaise, pneumonia, maculopapular rash and lymphadenopathy. Individuals can be infected only once and so a woman who is immune prior to pregnancy is not at risk of transmitting the organism to her infant. Serological tests are used to confirm the diagnosis, but their interpretation can be difficult, since latent infection is common. Demonstration of a rising titre of IgG-specific antibody or the presence of specific IgM antibody indicates active infection.

Infection during pregnancy can be transmitted to the fetus and the clinical manifestations of congenital toxoplasmosis, which include choroidoretinitis, recurrent seizures, hydrocephalus and intracranial calcifications may be present at birth or manifest later. The risk to the fetus is related to the gestation at which maternal infection occurs. Infection in the first trimester is less likely to be transmitted to the fetus (17%) and the risk of fetal infection is highest in the third trimester (65%). However, transmission in the first trimester is associated with spontaneous miscarriage and more severe symptoms in the neonate. The presence of hydrocephalus and scattered intracranial calcification, with a predilection for the basal ganglia, may be identified on ultrasound scan.

The prevalence of seropositivity, which indicates past infection and therefore immunity, and the risk of acquisition during pregnancy vary among countries, perhaps because of cultural differences in the handling of raw meat and the disposal of cat litter. Antenatal screening for toxoplasmosis is conducted in some countries, such as France, but not in the UK. In this country, pregnant women are advised to avoid emptying cat litter trays, to avoid contact with sick cats and to wear gloves when gardening. All meat should be cooked thoroughly and all surfaces and utensils should be washed after preparing raw meat.

The treatment of choice for toxoplasmosis infection is a combination of pyrimethamine and sulfadiazine given for several weeks. However, pyrimethamine is a folate antagonist and is theoretically teratogenic. It should therefore be avoided in the first trimester of pregnancy. When this combination is employed later in pregnancy, folic acid supplements should be given and full blood counts performed weekly. Spiramycin is a safer alternative during pregnancy and may reduce the risk of transmission of maternal infection to the fetus.

Cytomegalovirus

Cytomegalovirus (CMV) is the most common viral infection transmitted to the fetus *in utero*. About 40–50% of women in the UK are susceptible, of whom 1% will have CMV-infected babies. If the mother is infected during pregnancy, the chance that the fetus will be damaged is about 4%. Therefore, approximately 0.4% of UK children are congenitally infected but most do not suffer sequelae. Primary maternal infection is almost always asymptomatic and repeated serological tests have to be performed to make the diagnosis. Fetal infection can also follow viral reactivation.

The highest risk to the fetus is when infection occurs in the first trimester and this may result in miscarriage or congenital abnormality. Infection later in pregnancy can result in growth restriction, hydrocephalus, intracranial calcification and chorioretinitis. The diagnosis of maternal infection is confirmed by demonstrating CMV-specific IgM. Fetal infection can be confirmed by identifying the virus in specimens obtained at amniocentesis or chorion villus sampling, while ultrasound may detect growth restriction, microcephaly, hydrocephalus or intracranial calcification.

The majority of congenitally infected neonates are asymptomatic and diagnosis is by serum testing. While most of these children will develop normally, some exhibit neurological sequelae, including deafness and learning difficulties later in life. A small proportion of neonates display the symptoms and signs of severe generalised infection. These infants have jaundice, hepatosplenomegaly, thrombocytopenia and haemolytic anaemia which may lead to hydrops. Microcephaly and chorioretinitis may occur and surviving infants are usually deaf and mentally retarded. Unlike rubella infection, the fetus can be adversely affected by infection in any of the three trimesters of pregnancy.

Chlamydia trachomatis

Infection with *Chlamydia trachomatis* is important during pregnancy mainly because of the potential adverse effects of infection on the neonate. *Chlamydia trachomatis* is a sexually transmitted infection and is often asymptomatic in the mother. Some infected women may have mucopurulent cervicitis, salpingitis or the urethral syndrome. Vertical transmission can occur through contact with infected maternal genital tract secretions during delivery and may result in ophthalmia neonatorum or pneumonia in the neonate. The risk of the neonate developing moderate to severe conjunctivitis is about 15–25% and for pneumonia, 5–15%. Postpartum endometritis can result from chlamydial infection.

During pregnancy, the diagnosis of chlamydial infection is made by culture of the organism from endocervical secretions, identification of chlamydial antigens directly in endocervical smears or by means of the ligase chain reaction assay, which employs nucleic acid amplification and is more sensitive than tissue culture methods. Outwith pregnancy, the agents of choice for the treatment of *Chlamydia trachomatis* are the tetracyclines. However, these agents are contraindicated in pregnancy because they are associated with teeth and bone abnormalities in the fetus. Erythromycin is generally regarded as the drug of choice in pregnancy, although many women find this drug unpleasant to take because of its gastrointestinal effects. Recent studies have suggested that amoxycillin is an acceptable alternative therapy for the treatment of *Chlamydia trachomatis* infection in pregnancy. Treatment with azithromycin and clindamycin requires further evaluation.

Listeriosis

Infection with *Listeria monocytogenes* is uncommon but the organism has a predilection for pregnant women. Infection can occur at any time of pregnancy. In some women the infection is asymptomatic, being diagnosed retrospectively after an adverse pregnancy outcome. During the bacteraemic phase of the infection, the woman may experience a mild, flu-like illness with fever, headache, myalgia and back-pain, with occasional gastrointestinal symptoms. Symptoms may mimic urinary tract infection. Placental transfer of the infection may result in chorioamnionitis, spontaneous miscarriage, stillbirth, preterm labour or delivery of an infected infant. Contaminated food is the usual source of infection and pregnant women are advised to avoid eating all types of paté and ripened soft cheeses. Pregnant women should avoid cooked-chilled meals and ready-to-eat poultry, unless thoroughly reheated before they are eaten. High standards of food hygiene can also decrease infection.

Although listeriosis can be severe during pregnancy and can result in adult respiratory distress syndrome, the main concerns surround its effects on the pregnancy. Listeriosis may result in:

- congenital listeriosis following transplacental passage of the organism
- mid-trimester pregnancy loss and preterm labour
- perinatal listeriosis which has early and late onset forms.

Treatment of maternal and neonatal infection is with high doses of intravenous antibiotics; ampicillin and gentamicin, high-dose penicillin or trimethoprim-sulphamethoxazole have each been used.

(V) ANAEMIA

Physiology

The diagnosis of anaemia is altered in pregnancy due to normal physiological changes in plasma and blood volume. By 32 weeks of gestation, the plasma volume has increased by around 50% with a concomitant increase in red cell mass of the order of 25%. In view of the relatively greater increase in plasma volume, the haemoglobin concentration, red-cell count and haematocrit will fall due to dilution. These changes will be exaggerated in multiple pregnancy when there are larger increases in the plasma volume. There should be no change in the mean corpuscular volume (MCV) or mean corpuscular haemoglobin concentration (MCHC). The maternal requirement for iron increases during pregnancy by two- to three-fold and the folate requirements by ten- to twenty-fold.

Ideally, the haemoglobin should not fall below 10.5 g/dl during pregnancy. The most common form of anaemia in pregnancy is iron deficiency anaemia. Deficiency of folic acid may co-exist along with iron deficiency, particularly as both can be associated with poor diet. If folic acid and iron are both deficient, the effects of folic acid deficiency are masked by iron deficiency. Folic acid deficiency may be caused by the administration of anticonvulsant medication. Vitamin B12 deficiency is rare in pregnancy.

Diagnosis of anaemia

The diagnosis of anaemia during pregnancy is usually made on routine testing of the full blood count, either at booking or in the third trimester. In severe cases it may be symptomatic and present with tiredness, dizziness, lethargy, fainting or dyspnoea, although these symptoms are not uncommon in normal pregnancy.

The main diagnostic criteria are the red cell indices on the full blood count. In iron deficiency anaemia, the MCV, MCHC and mean cell haemoglobin (MCH) are all reduced. Consideration should be given to the differential diagnosis of thalassaemia, which shows a reduced MCV and MCH but normal or only slightly reduced MCHC. The blood film in classic iron deficiency anaemia shows hypochromic microcytic red cells just as in the nonpregnant condition. However, this characteristic red cell morphology occurs relatively late in the development of the anaemia and will be preceded by a reduction in the MCV and, subsequently, a reduction in the MCHC. Indeed, a woman can be deficient in iron and present with a normochromic, normocytic anaemia. In the situation where the red cell indices are not diagnostic of iron deficiency anaemia, serum ferritin is the most useful measure of iron status with a concentration of serum ferritin of less than 12 µg/l being compatible with iron deficiency. In the normal situation, serum ferritin falls over the course of a pregnancy and this requires to be taken into account in the interpretation of serum ferritin results. Although the serum iron and total iron-binding capacity (TIBC) fall in normal pregnancy, a serum iron less than 12 µmol/l and a TIBC saturation less than 15% indicate iron deficiency. Since the serum iron and TIBC can fluctuate widely during pregnancy and are affected by iron ingestion, they are less helpful in diagnosis than serum ferritin. Folic acid deficiency causes a macrocytic anaemia with a raised MCV. The diagnosis is confirmed by finding a reduced serum and red cell folate.

With improvements in living standards and nutrition, a tendency for women to have fewer children and hormonal contraception reducing menstrual blood loss, the incidence of anaemia in pregnancy has declined over the past fifty years. In parallel, there has been a trend for women not to be given routine iron or folic acid supplements during pregnancy. Despite this, some clinicians propose that routine iron and folate supplementation should continue, since many women still enter pregnancy with reduced iron stores and the increased demands for iron during pregnancy cannot be met by increased absorption alone. Further, the benefit of preconceptual and first-trimester folic acid (0.4 mg/day) in the prevention of neural tube defects is well recognised.

The usual treatment of iron-deficiency anaemia is oral iron supplementation, which should be combined with folic acid supplements. Concurrent administration of vitamin C (50 mg or greater with each dose of iron sulphate) may enhance the absorption of iron as well as being important for red cell production. Parenteral iron therapy (intramuscular or intravenous) is rarely required and should only be used where there is serious intolerance of oral iron. With appropriate correction of iron deficiency the haemoglobin should increase by between 0.8 g/dl and 1 g/dl per week. Parenteral administration does not correct the iron deficiency more rapidly. In women close to term who are profoundly anaemic, blood transfusion may be required to increase the haemoglobin before delivery.

(VI) CONNECTIVE TISSUE DISEASE

The main connective tissue diseases seen in pregnancy are rheumatoid arthritis and systemic lupus erythematosus.

Rheumatoid arthritis

Rheumatoid arthritis is an autoimmune disorder causing chronic inflammation of, primarily, the synovial joints. It complicates about one in every 1500 pregnancies but rarely causes significant problems since the disease often improves (75%) during the course of the pregnancy. This may be due to an increased concentration of anti-inflammatory steroid hormones. A large proportion (up to 90%) of those women who experience an improvement in symptoms during pregnancy will experience a postpartum flare.

The main concern for women with rheumatoid arthritis during pregnancy is the effect of drug treatments on the fetus. Fortunately, in many women, an improvement in symptoms means that analgesic and anti-inflammatory requirements can be reduced or discontinued during pregnancy. Simple analgesics such as paracetamol may be used freely in pregnancy. Nonsteroidal anti-inflammatory drugs (NSAIDs) can also be used, although there are concerns regarding the effects of these agents on the fetus. Chronic use of NSAIDs may result in oligohydramnios due to suppressed fetal urine production and, occasionally, when used in the third trimester, premature closure of the ductus arteriosis which may in turn place the fetus at risk of pulmonary hypertension. These agents can inhibit neonatal platelet function, thereby increasing the risk of haemorrhage. Thus, the use of such agents should be limited as much as possible and ideally should be discontinued in the third trimester (Table 7.10). Corticosteroid therapy is safe in pregnancy and can be used to control symptoms in the third trimester when NSAIDs are contraindicated.

Corticosteroids are not teratogenic but prolonged use during pregnancy is associated with intrauterine growth restriction. Chronic administration is associated with gestational diabetes, maternal osteoporosis and an elevation in maternal blood pressure and will also result in the need for steroid supplements during labour (usually 100–150 mg hydrocortisone intravenously six to eight hourly). Although uncommon, fetal adrenal suppression may also occur with high doses and prolonged maternal therapy; the neonate may occasionally require steroid supplements following delivery. Other agents employed in the management of rheumatoid arthritis are shown in Table 7.10.

Systemic lupus erythematosus

In contrast to rheumatoid arthritis, systemic lupus erythematosus (SLE) is associated with particular problems in pregnancy. SLE affects about one in 1000 women and is most commonly diagnosed in the child-

Table 7.10 Drug treatments for rheumatoid arthritis in pregnancy

Drug	Comments
Paracetamol	First-line agent
Non-steroidal anti-inflammatory drugs	Should be avoided in the late third trimester; liquor volume should be monitored during their use
Corticosteroids	Preferable to non-steroidal anti-inflammatory drugs in the third trimester
Azathioprine	Appears to be safe, although long-term fetal effects unknown
D-penicillamine	May be teratogenic (avoid)
Gold salts	Teratogenic in animals (avoid)
Antimalarials	High doses associated with fetal retinopathy and should only be used if the disease is not otherwise controlled
Sulfasalazine	No adverse effects known in pregnancy, although it antagonises folic acid (hence give folic acid supplements)
Antimitotic agents	Contraindicated in pregnancy

bearing years (25–35 years). This autoimmune condition produces specific cytotoxic antibodies provoking problems such as haemolytic anaemia or thrombocytopenia and immune complex problems associated with inflammatory lesions affecting the kidneys, the skin and the central nervous system. The major immune complex implicated is DNA-anti-DNA. Arthritis is a common manifestation (90%) of SLE and is usually non-deforming, in contrast to the arthritis found in rheumatoid arthritis. Evidence of chronic glomerulonephritis is present in over 50% of women with SLE. Disease activity can be assessed by the presence of anti-native DNA antibodies and depressed levels of the complement components, C3 and C4.

EFFECT OF SLE ON PREGNANCY

SLE is associated with a number of adverse outcomes in pregnancy (Table 7.11). Miscarriage is more common, occurring in between 28 and 40% of pregnancies. The incidence is even higher (up to 60%) in women who have anticardiolipin antibodies and antibodies directed against cytoplasmic ribonucleoprotein Ro (anti-Ro). There is an increase in

Table 7.11 Maternal and fetal risks associated with systemic lupus erythematosus

	Risk
Maternal	Flare up of disease, particularly in early pregnancy and postpartum Pre-eclampsia Deterioration in renal function Arterial and venous thrombotic problems (including deep vein thrombosis and cerebral thrombosis) often associated with lupus anticoagulant and anticardiolipin antibodies
Fetal and neonatal	Spontaneous miscarriage Intrauterine death (due to problems such as growth restriction and placental infarction) Prematurity (iatrogenic or spontaneous) Intrauterine growth restriction (may be associated with pre-eclampsia) Congenital heart block and cardiac failure (associated with anti-Ro antibodies) Neonatal lupus

perinatal mortality and an increase in the incidence of intrauterine growth restriction (20%), pre-eclampsia (25–30%) and preterm delivery (25–60%).

EFFECT OF PREGNANCY ON SLE

The reported risk of a flare in disease activity during pregnancy varies with the population studied and the type of study performed. Most of the reported controlled studies do indicate that a flare is more likely to occur during pregnancy with a relative risk of about 2.5. Overall, about 15% of women experience a flare during pregnancy with renal and haematological involvement being more common, and joint involvement less common.

PREPREGNANCY COUNSELLING

In view of the maternal and fetal risks associated with SLE (Table 7.11), prepregnancy counselling is important in the management of these woman. This will allow the patient to determine on an informed basis whether or not to become pregnant. She should be advised that it is optimal for her to conceive while the disease is quiescent and where drug therapy is minimal. Her blood pressure should be measured and her renal function determined. Hydroxychloroquine may have adverse effects on the fetal retina and should, if possible, be discontinued before conception. If the woman conceives on hydroxychloroquine, then she should continue this treatment since stopping may result in a flare. Azathiaprine should be avoided if possible but if it is required for disease control then it should not be withheld. Corticosteroids can be used safely in pregnancy with no evidence of teratogenicity in the human, although their use is associated with fetal intrauterine growth restriction. However, the overriding interest in SLE is quiescent disease and, thus, steroid administration to the mother should not be withheld. In the prepregnancy situation she should be reassured with regard to the effects of steroids on the pregnancy.

It is also worth assessing not only disease activity but also for the presence of anticardiolipin antibodies and lupus anticoagulant in prepregnancy as well as the presence or absence of anti-Ro antibody. Anti-Ro antibodies are present in less than 1% of the general population but 30% of patients with SLE. However, should the lupus anticoagulant and anticardiolipin antibody results be negative it is often worthwhile repeating them during pregnancy as sometimes anticardiolipin antibodies are only evident in the course of a pregnancy. The presence of anti-Ro antibodies places the patient at increased risk of congenital heart block as these antibodies cross the placenta and attack the conducting system of the developing fetal heart (see below).

ANTENATAL MANAGEMENT

Women with SLE should be managed jointly by obstetricians with a particular interest in medical disorders and rheumatologists. In view of the numerous fetal risks associated with SLE it is usual to prescribe prophylactic low-dose aspirin at a dose of 75 mg from the end of the first trimester or earlier should there be a history of miscarriage or previous problems. Some clinicians advocate that women with SLE should commence low-dose aspirin prior to conception since the placental damage in SLE occurs early in pregnancy. Low-dose aspirin is not associated with adverse maternal or fetal affects and thus can be used safely throughout pregnancy. The policy at Glasgow Royal Infirmary is to start treatment with low-dose aspirin when the woman first presents in pregnancy and to commence it prior to pregnancy in women with recurrent miscarriage. It is continued throughout pregnancy, in view of the potential for late pregnancy problems for mother and baby.

Where anticardiolipin antibodies or lupus anticoagulant are found then thromboprophylaxis must be implemented. Where a patient has such antibodies and a past history of thrombosis or recurrent miscarriage, it would be usual to prescribe low-dose unfractionated or low-molecular-weight heparin through the pregnancy together with low-dose aspirin. In any event, postpartum thromboprophylaxis should be used as there may be substantial risk of venous thromboembolic disease in the puerperium. Postpartum thromboprophylaxis should usually be continued for at least six weeks and unfractionated or low-molecular-weight heparin can be used in this situation. The Glasgow Royal Infirmary policy of thromboprophylaxis during pregnancy for women with anticardiolipin antibodies is outlined in Table 7.12.

Careful maternal and fetal monitoring is required through the pregnancy. Early in pregnancy, the gestation should be accurately determined and, at 18 and 24 weeks of gestation, maternal uterine artery Doppler studies should be performed and may identify women at increased risk of adverse perinatal outcome. Fetal growth should be monitored fortnightly from 26 weeks of gestation by serial ultrasound scans and umbilical artery flow velocity waveforms assessed using Doppler ultrasound are also of value in identifying fetuses at high risk from growth restriction. Assessment of fetal well-being should be undertaken from the late second trimester using ultrasound scanning (biophysical profile scoring and/or umbilical artery Doppler studies) and cardiotocography. The intensity of monitoring for fetal well-being will depend on the presence of complications such as growth restriction.

Table 7.12 Antenatal thromboprophylaxis in pregnancy for women with anticardiolipin antibodies (ACA)

Patient	Thromboprophylaxis
Asymptomatic woman with ACA	Low-dose aspirin
ACA and recurrent miscarriage	Low-dose aspirin and low-molecular-weight heparin
ACA and previous IUGR or pre-eclampsia	Low-dose aspirin and consider low-molecular-weight heparin
ACA and previous venous thromboembolism	Low-dose aspirin and low-molecular-weight heparin (may require therapeutic doses, if normally on warfarin)

Maternal monitoring is aimed at detecting flare-up of lupus, any deterioration in renal function and the development of superimposed pre-eclampsia. It is often difficult to determine whether the onset of problems such as oedema, hypertension and proteinuria are due to superimposed pre-eclampsia or a flare-up of lupus nephritis. The occurrence of these manifestations in the absence of other evidence of a flare-up in SLE and in the absence of serologic abnormalities suggests superimposed pre-eclampsia. Elevated DNA antibodies and suppressed complement levels would favour the diagnosis of flare in SLE. Should a flare-up of SLE occur it would be usual to treat the patient initially with corticosteroids. Hypertension should be treated with methyldopa, nifedipine or labetalol.

Timing and mode of delivery will depend on the development of any complications. When significant fetal compromise is present it is usual to perform caesarean section. Steroid supplements will be needed to cover both labour and caesarean section.

NEONATAL LUPUS

The treatment of SLE in pregnancy requires a multi-disciplinary approach, which should include a neonatologist. Antibodies directed against cytoplasmic ribonucleoproteins Ro and La can cross the placenta and have adverse effects on the fetus. The most common effect is cutaneous neonatal lupus, which occurs in 5% of neonates whose mothers have anti-Ro antibodies. It presents as a characteristic rash on the face and scalp in the first two weeks of life and normally resolves within six months. Congenital heart block occurs in about 3% of neonates of Ro-positive mothers and, in contrast to cutaneous lupus, develops *in utero*. This is thought to arise from damage to the fetal heart conducting system and can usually be detected by the end of the second trimester on detailed ultrasound scanning. This problem is not reversible and the babies born with congenital heart block will have this as a persistent problem through their life. Cardiac failure can develop *in utero*, leading to hydrops and fetal death, and may respond to salbutamol, dexamethasone or plasmapheresis. These treatments will, however, have no effect on the damaged conducting system. When congenital heart block is detected *in utero*, delivery should be by caesarean section since the fetus is less able to deal with the stress of labour; fetal heart rate monitoring is not possible during labour. About 30% of neonates born with congenital heart block will die in the early neonatal period and the majority of survivors will require pacemakers.

Lupus anticoagulant and anticardiolipin antibody syndrome

Lupus anticoagulant and anticardiolipin antibodies occur in 5–20% of patients with SLE. However, these antibodies can commonly occur in patients without underlying SLE, with only around 50% of patients with anticardiolipin antibodies and lupus anticoagulant having underlying SLE.

Lupus anticoagulant is an IgG or IgM antibody against phospholipids which interferes with the activation of prothrombin by the prothrombin converting complex of factor Va and factor Xa, calcium and lipid. A variety of laboratory tests are used to determine the presence of lupus anticoagulant; in particular, the activated partial thromboplastin time, the dilute prothrombin time and the Russell's viper venom time. There is prolongation of these coagulation tests in the laboratory. The name lupus anticoagulant reflects the association with SLE and the prolongation of the coagulation tests *in vitro*. Despite this, *in vivo* problems relate to thrombosis, which can occur at the level of the placental bed, so triggering problems such as growth restriction, placental infarction and fetal death, and arterial and venous thromboembolic events as noted above.

Anticardiolipin antibodies are antibodies specifically directed against phospholipids in cell membranes. They often co-exist with lupus anticoagulant but they are not one and the same. High levels of anticardiolipin antibodies are powerful predictors of fetal compromise and are associated with a high risk of fetal death in women with SLE. These antibodies have also been associated with recurrent miscarriage, growth restriction and increased risk of pre-eclampsia, as well as arterial and venous thrombotic events as noted above. Patients with lupus anticoagulant and anticardiolipin antibodies are usually treated with low-dose aspirin 75 mg once a day in an attempt to prevent these thrombotic complications. In patients with a history of thrombotic problems or recurrent miscarriage, aspirin is combined with antenatal thromboprophylaxis with subcutaneous unfractionated or low-molecular-weight heparin. The addition of steroids to aspirin or heparin is not usually warranted. Steroids should only be used in patients with active SLE where steroids would be required in any event. Patients with a history of unexplained fetal loss, growth restriction, severe pre-eclampsia or recurrent miscarriage should be screened for anticardiolipin antibodies and lupus anticoagulant.

(VII) MALIGNANCY

Malignancy is among the major causes of non-accidental death in women of childbearing age in the developed world and it has been estimated that one in 1000 women will be affected by malignancy during pregnancy. For women aged 15–34 years, the most common malignancies are cervical cancer, breast cancer, leukaemia, central nervous system tumours and non-Hodgkin lymphoma. In women aged 35–54 years, lung, colorectal and ovarian cancer also become common malignancies. This section will consider only the two most common malignancies associated with pregnancy, namely cervical and breast cancer.

Cervical cancer

The most common malignancy associated with pregnancy is invasive carcinoma of the cervix. The incidence of this disease has declined from 1/2200 pregnancies in the 1970s to 1.2/10 000 pregnancies in the 1980s. This reduction may be due to the implementation of adequate cervical screening programmes. Current literature indicates that maternal survival and tumour behaviour are not influenced by pregnancy. In general, when invasive carcinoma of the cervix is diagnosed in the first and early second trimesters, therapeutic termination is offered and immediate treatment commenced. When the fetus is viable a delay in definitive treatment to allow for fetal maturity can be contemplated.

Breast cancer

Carcinoma of the breast is the second most common malignancy associated with pregnancy, complicating approximately 1/3000 to 1/10 000 pregnancies. Pregnant women with breast cancer are more likely to be diagnosed with advanced disease and their overall survival is lower than nonpregnant controls. This may be due to physiological changes of the breasts during pregnancy obscuring any masses and therefore delaying diagnosis. Also, some clinicians are reluctant to biopsy breast lumps during pregnancy. Mammography is less sensitive in detecting malignancy during pregnancy. When matched for stage of disease, there is no difference in survival.

There appears to be no survival benefit from termination of pregnancy and subsequent pregnancy after treated disease does not alter the outcome. Breast cancer diagnosed during pregnancy is associated with preterm delivery and intrauterine growth restriction. Treatment of the disease, the cancer itself or the stress of the diagnosis may cause this latter effect. The current literature on the use of chemotherapy in pregnant women with breast cancer is sparse and in the form of case reports. Radiotherapy for breast cancer is avoided during pregnancy since the therapeutic doses of radiation used result in significant exposure of the fetus.

Chemotherapy during pregnancy

The risk of teratogenesis following exposure to chemotherapeutic agents in the first trimester is well documented. In a review of 169 women treated with chemotherapy for various malignancies in the first trimester, Doll et al. (1988) reported a 25% rate of fetal abnormality following combination therapy and 17% for single-agent treatment. When those women who received concomitant radiotherapy or folate antagonists were excluded, the incidence of fetal abnormality following single-agent chemotherapy was only 6%. Following exposure to chemotherapeutic agents in the second and third trimesters, the rate of malformations was only 1.5%. Zemlickis et al. (1992) reported the outcomes of 21 pregnancies in women who had received chemotherapy for various cancers. Of these 21 women, 13 received their chemotherapy in the first trimester. Five of these pregnancies progressed to term and two of the five had major malformations: these infants were affected by intrauterine growth restriction and preterm delivery, compared with a control group. Of the remaining eight pregnancies, four were terminated therapeutically and four miscarried spontaneously. Long-term follow-up studies of children exposed to chemotherapy *in utero* are favourable, with normal intelligence quotient testing, physical development and haematological investigations.

References

Doll, D.C., Ringenberg, Q.S. and Yarbro, J.W. (1988) Management of cancer during pregnancy. *Arch Intern Med* **148**, 2058–64

Zemlickis, D., Lishner, M., Degendorfer, P. *et al*. (1992) Fetal outcome after *in utero* exposure to cancer chemotherapy. *Arch Intern Med* **152**, 573–6

(VIII) RESPIRATORY DISEASE

Physiological changes in the respiratory system in pregnancy

During pregnancy, oxygen consumption increases by up to around 30% because of the demands of the fetoplacental unit and an increased maternal metabolic rate. This is accompanied by increased production of CO_2. Despite this, arterial oxygen tensions are maintained within essentially normal nonpregnant limits, while carbon dioxide tension (Pa_{CO_2})

is reduced around 25% below the nonpregnant level. These changes are brought about by an increase in tidal volume of around 40% over baseline with little change in respiratory rate. In the third trimester the functional residual capacity is decreased. These physiological changes appear to be due to increased progesterone sensitising the respiratory centre and women often complain of dyspnoea in early pregnancy if they are aware of these changes. The decreased $Paco_2$ results in a compensatory fall in serum bicarbonate and, thus, a mild respiratory alkalosis is normal during pregnancy.

Asthma

Asthma is the most common chronic disease affecting children and young adults and it is becoming more common. Population studies indicate that up to 5% of pregnant women may be asthmatic. Some women may enter pregnancy with symptoms of chronic cough, wheeze and breathlessness, which they have come to accept as normal. Pregnancy therefore provides an opportunity to diagnose asthma and to provide appropriate treatment. The diagnosis is suggested by obtaining a history of typical symptoms, of which nocturnal wheezing or dyspnoea may be the most significant. Confirmation of the diagnosis may be made by recording an improvement of over 15% in the peak expiratory flow rate or forced expiratory volume in one second, after inhalation of a beta-sympathomimetic bronchodilator.

EFFECT OF PREGNANCY ON ASTHMA

Pregnancy does not have a consistent effect on asthma. In some women the asthma worsens and in others it stays the same and there are still others in whom the condition improves. The response is also not predictable between pregnancies. It would be unusual for a patient with well-controlled asthma and minimal symptoms to develop significant problems due to the enlarging uterus in the third trimester. However, pregnancy is normally associated with an increase in tidal volume, which may be interpreted as breathlessness. In addition, many women may adjust their therapy or even discontinue it if they are worried about the effects of drugs in pregnancy. Those women whose asthma improves during the third trimester may experience an exacerbation in symptoms postnatally.

EFFECT OF ASTHMA ON PREGNANCY

Well-controlled asthma is unlikely to have any adverse effects on the pregnancy and women should be advised of this and encouraged to continue with their medication. Uncontrolled severe asthma can be associated with significant maternal hypoxia, which could in turn have adverse consequences for the fetus. The drugs commonly used to treat asthma, including betasympathomimetics, inhaled and oral steroids, sodium cromoglycate and methyl xanthines, are not associated with teratogenesis or serious risk to the fetus. Where theophyllines are used, it should be noted that there is substantially increased renal clearance of the drug in pregnancy, making it more difficult to control, and drug levels should be monitored. Glasgow Royal Infirmary practice is to discontinue these and manage the patient as in Table 7.13. In patients on high-dose steroid therapy in the third trimester there is a small risk of a degree of suppression of the fetal hypothalamo-pituitary-adrenal axis and the patient should be warned of this in the event of the neonate requiring steroid supplements. In addition, the mother will be at risk of the usual adverse effects of steroids, including osteoporosis, weight gain, hypertension and gestational diabetes.

A number of studies have reported associations between maternal asthma and complications of pregnancy. Many of these studies have been criticised for their design or size. In summary, these studies have indicated a slight increase in preterm labour, intrauterine growth restriction, hypertensive disorders, and an increased neonatal morbidity in women with asthma.

Management

PREPREGNANCY

When the asthmatic patient is seen prior to conception, her treatment should be optimised and she should be reassured that her medication will not influence the outcome of the pregnancy. Further, she should be advised that the effects of uncontrolled asthma pose a greater risk to the pregnancy. It should be emphasised that good control of her asthma is critically important to her pregnancy.

ANTENATAL MANAGEMENT

Treatment of asthma during pregnancy is the same as treatment in non-pregnant subjects (Table 7.13). The aim of treatment is to prevent attacks and to provide the woman with a symptom-free lifestyle. Treatment can be assessed by home monitoring of peak flow levels. If there are any triggering factors, such as exposure to pollens, then clearly these should be avoided if possible. For mildly affected individuals with symptoms once each day, the use of an inhaled betasympathomimetic, such as salbutamol or terbutaline, is satisfactory. If more frequent symptoms

Table 7.13 Treatment of asthma in pregnancy

Step	Treatment
1	Occasional use of short-acting betasympathomimetic bronchodilators (salbutamol or terbutaline)
2	Inhaled short-acting betasympathomimetics as required PLUS Regular inhaled anti-inflammatory agents (beclomethasone or budesonide, 100–400 µg twice daily)
3	Inhaled short-acting betasympathomimetics as required High-dose inhaled steroids (800–2000 µg of beclomethasone or budesonide daily) OR Steroid inhalers as Step 2 plus salmeterol (long-acting bronchodilator 50 mg twice daily)
4	Inhaled short-acting betasympathomimetics as required High-dose steroid inhalers as Step 3 PLUS Sequential trials of additional therapy, e.g. ipratropium, sodium cromoglycate or high-dose inhaled bronchodilators
5	Inhaled short-acting betasympathomimetics as required High-dose inhaled steroid as in Step 3 PLUS One or more long-acting bronchodilators PLUS Regular prednisolone in single daily dose (steroid supplements will be required in labour or with caesarean section)

occur, regular use of a steroid inhaler should be employed with intermittent inhaled beta-agonists as required. Where symptoms are not controlled with this therapy, high-dose inhaled steroids may be required and the addition of a long-acting betasympathomimetic such as salmeterol may be of value. In the most severe cases, systemic corticosteroids would be required.

Animal studies have suggested that systemic corticosteroids are associated with an increased incidence of cleft palate and these studies were inappropriately extrapolated to human pregnancy. It is now accepted that systemic corticosteroids are not teratogenic in humans. However, they can be associated with intrauterine growth restriction and fetal growth should be assessed by ultrasound in the third trimester. Further, they increase the risk of gestational diabetes and maternal blood glucose should be assessed regularly and a glucose tolerance test performed if indicated. When systemic corticosteroids have been taken regularly it would be usual to cover delivery with intravenous hydrocortisone 100–150 mg intravenously every six to eight hours during labour. Rarely, the fetal adrenal gland may be suppressed following delivery.

Asthma is usually worse during the night and early morning. Hence, women seen at the antenatal clinic during working hours should be asked about symptoms producing sleep disturbance. Women with wide diurnal swings on peak flow testing are at greatest risk of acute deterioration. Acute severe asthma can be extremely dangerous and should be managed aggressively in hospital. Admission to the intensive care unit may be required for severe asthma during pregnancy. A failure to respond to vigorous management (rehydration, oxygen, nebulised beta-sympathomimetics and steroids orally and intravenously), should suggest concurrent pathology, including pulmonary thromboembolism.

Any suspicion of infection, which often precipitates an acute attack, should be properly treated with antibiotics. The usual antibiotics can be prescribed for chest infection in pregnancy with the exception of tetracyclines, which should be avoided because of their effect on fetal bones and teeth. As there is a substantial increase in the clearance of the penicillins during pregnancy, the dose of ampicillin or amoxycillin should be doubled for systemic infections.

INTRAPARTUM MANAGEMENT

Prophylactic treatment should continue during labour. Although oral and intravenous betasympathomimetics are often employed as tocolytic agents during pregnancy, there is no evidence that inhaled betasympathomimetics impair uterine activity or delay the onset of labour. During induction of labour some caution should be exercised with prostaglandin agents used for cervical ripening, particularly prostaglandin F_2 which causes bronchospasm. Prostaglandin E_2 is a bronchodilator and can be used safely in these women. General anaesthesia should be avoided for operative delivery, if possible, and for women with severe disease an anaesthetic review should be arranged in the third trimester. Ergometrine should not be used for the third stage of labour since it can cause bronchospasm; oxytocin alone should therefore be used.

Postpartum, the woman should continue her therapy and breastfeeding is not contraindicated. Physiotherapy may be required, especially if an operative delivery has occurred. Pulmonary function may be impaired due to a surgical wound or a degree of atelectasis following a general anaesthetic.

Tuberculosis

The incidence of tuberculosis is on the increase and it may be associated with HIV infection. In the UK, it is more common in Asian and West Indian families. It is essential that tuberculosis in pregnancy is treated by a respiratory physician or an infectious-diseases physician. The diagnosis of tuberculosis during pregnancy should be borne in mind in women presenting with weight loss or failure to gain weight, nocturnal sweats, cough and haemoptysis. A chest X-ray should not be withheld during pregnancy when it is clinically indicated and sputum should be sent for examination for acid-fast tubercle bacilli. When sputum samples cannot be obtained, fibre optic bronchoscopy should be arranged and washings sent for tubercle examination.

When tuberculosis is diagnosed after the first trimester, treatment should follow established guidelines with combination chemotherapy with pyrazinamide, rifampicin and isoniazid for two months, followed by a further four months of rifampicin and isoniazid. Pyridoxine (50 mg/day) should be given together with isoniazid to reduce the risk of peripheral neuritis. There is some concern over the use of this regimen in the first trimester. While ethambutol and isoniazid are considered safe for the fetus, there are concerns with regard to both rifampicin and streptomycin, the latter having been shown to have a high incidence (over 10%) of VIII nerve damage. Teratogenic effects have been reported with rifampicin in animal studies, although there is no convincing evidence for these effects in humans. Many clinicians now regard this drug to be safe in the first trimester. There is limited experience of the use of pyrazinamide in pregnancy. Thus, in patients who present in the first trimester, it may be best to avoid streptomycin, pyrazinamide and perhaps also rifampicin. If possible, treat the patient with isoniazid and ethambutol alone, moving on to the triple therapy in the second trimester. Where a patient is seriously ill with tuberculosis in the first trimester, pyrazinamide or rifampicin should be employed as required.

Infection with tuberculosis does not seem to have adverse effects upon the pregnancy, nor does pregnancy alter disease progression in women who receive adequate anti-tuberculous treatment. Extra-pulmonary tuberculosis is usually not infectious. Patients with pulmonary tuberculosis who are not coughing sputum or where the sputum has been shown not to contain tubercle bacilli should be regarded as non-infectious. Patients whose pulmonary sputum is positive are infectious, although treatment will usually result in them becoming non-infectious within around two weeks. Congenital tuberculosis resulting from transfer of bacilli across the placenta or from amniotic fluid or secretions during delivery is rare. The neonate is at risk of airborne infection if the mother has active tuberculosis at the time of delivery. Where the neonate is considered at risk it should be immunised with isoniazid-resistant BCG injection and concomitant isoniazid. Women should be reassured that they can breastfeed during treatment with antituberculous medication.

(IX) GASTROINTESTINAL DISEASE AND HEPATIC DISEASE

Physiological changes during pregnancy

Gastrointestinal motility is reduced during pregnancy, with delayed gastric emptying and reduced bowel transit times. There is a reduction in distal oesophageal pressure. These changes mean that heartburn, nausea, vomiting and constipation are common during normal pregnancy. There is an increase in liver metabolism during pregnancy. Alkaline phosphatase rises during pregnancy, mainly due to production by the placenta, but the other liver enzymes are largely unchanged.

Reflux oesophagitis

Oesophagitis arises from reflux of gastric contents into the lower oesophagus, which results in inflammation. This is extremely common because of the reduction in lower oesophageal pressure and delayed gastric emptying during pregnancy. The enlarging gravid uterus exacerbates the condition in late pregnancy. Reflux most commonly presents with heartburn, nausea and vomiting. Less often, the woman with reflux will present with haematemesis or respiratory symptoms. The pharmacological management of reflux includes antacid preparations, the histamine-receptor antagonist ranitidine, metoclopramide and sucralfate. Postural changes, particularly at night with elevation of the head of the bed, and dietary modifications may be helpful.

Peptic ulcer disease

Peptic ulcer disease is traditionally thought to occur less commonly during pregnancy. This may be explained by a protective effect of pregnancy-induced prostaglandins on the gastric mucosa. Alternatively, the incidence of peptic ulcer disease during pregnancy may be underestimated because of a reluctance to perform endoscopy during pregnancy and an eagerness on the part of clinicians to ascribe symptoms to reflux. The presenting symptoms of peptic ulcer disease include epigastric pain, nausea and vomiting; gastrointestinal haemorrhage and perforation are extremely uncommon during pregnancy. The diagnosis is confirmed by endoscopy, which can be performed during pregnancy and is indicated when epigastric pain complicates nausea, vomiting and heartburn. The management includes antacids, ranitidine and sucralfate. When peptic ulcers have remained quiescent during pregnancy, a postpartum exacerbation in symptoms is not uncommon.

It is critical that epigastric pain in pregnancy is never attributed to a gastrointestinal problem until pre-eclampsia has been excluded.

Inflammatory bowel disease

Inflammatory bowel disease (Crohn's disease and ulcerative colitis) tends to present in young adulthood (20–40 years), and has an incidence of approximately 10 per 100 000. Crohn's disease can affect any part of the gastrointestinal tract but has a particular tendency to affect the terminal ileum, while ulcerative colitis is always confined to the colon. There is overlap between these two conditions in their clinical, histological and radiological features.

Most women with inflammatory bowel disease find that pregnancy has little effect on the course of their disease. The outcome is best if their disease is quiescent at the time of conception. Exacerbation of ulcerative colitis tends to occur in the first half of pregnancy, while increased disease activity in Crohn's most commonly presents in the first trimester. Exacerbation is more common in women who conceive during periods of active disease activity and a postpartum flare may occur with Crohn's disease.

For the majority of women, the disease has no effect on their pregnancy. Active disease early in pregnancy is associated with spontaneous miscarriage and, later in pregnancy, with an increased risk of preterm delivery. Delivery by caesarean section should be reserved for obstetric indications, for women with perianal Crohn's and those with a history of extensive surgery. Where an ileo-anal anastomosis and pouch is in place, delivery should be by caesarean section. Women who have previously undergone surgical management cope well with pregnancy and labour, although transient ileostomy dysfunction may occur from midpregnancy. This often resolves with fasting and intravenous fluids. Acute inflammatory bowel disease is an important risk factor for venous thromboembolism. Thrombotic risk should be considered and thromboprophylaxis instituted where multiple risk factors are present.

Prepregnancy counselling is important, since women should be encouraged to postpone conception until their disease is quiescent. Disease activity during pregnancy can be managed with sulphasalazine and corticosteroids given orally and by enema. Folic acid supplements should be given with sulphasalazine. When complications of the disease arise (perforation, obstruction, abscess formation and toxic megacolon), surgery may be required.

Intrahepatic cholestasis of pregnancy

Intrahepatic cholestasis of pregnancy (ICP, also known as obstetric cholestasis) is associated with an increased incidence of adverse maternal and fetal outcome. The prevalence of the condition in the UK is 0.5–1%, although it may be as high as 12% in certain populations, such as Chile. The pathogenesis of ICP is incompletely understood although there appears to be a genetic predisposition to the cholestatic effect of elevated circulating oestrogen. The clinical presentation of ICP includes generalised, severe pruritus often associated with dark urine and pale stools. Liver function tests are abnormal, with elevated transaminases, gamma-glutamyl transpeptidase and alkaline phosphatase. Bilirubin may be mildly elevated and the serum total bile acid concentration is increased.

Fetal associations with ICP include spontaneous preterm labour, intracranial haemorrhage, meconium staining, intrauterine fetal death and intrapartum fetal distress. Older series have reported a stillbirth rate of about 10%, although more recent series, where women were electively delivered by 38 weeks of gestation, indicate that this rate has reduced to 1–2%. However, there has been little change in the reported rates of preterm labour (30–40%) and meconium staining (25–35%). There is no evidence that regular assessment of fetal well-being, using cardiotocography and ultrasound Doppler studies, can prevent fetal distress or intrauterine death. The use of amniocentesis to detect meconium has been employed by some clinicians. The maternal risks of ICP include vitamin K deficiency (with subsequent disturbed coagulation) and an increased risk of antepartum haemorrhage. Further, these women have a significant risk (35%) of pruritis on combined oral contraceptives.

The management of ICP is to establish the diagnosis by excluding other causes of cholestasis (including viral hepatitis, gallstones and primary biliary cirrhosis) and then to counsel the mother about the adverse sequelae that are associated with the condition. Liver function tests and a coagulation screen should be assessed at least weekly and it may be useful to monitor bile acids. Antihistamines, cholestyramine and dexamethasone may relieve pruritis. Ursodeoxycholic acid, which has been used widely outwith pregnancy, may be of value in reducing serum bile acids, although experience with this agent during pregnancy is limited at present. The mother should be given vitamin K to reduce the risks of maternal and fetal haemorrhage. While the benefits of fetal surveillance are uncertain, most units perform cardiotocography and ultrasound scans for amniotic fluid volume, fetal growth, biophysical profile scores and Doppler studies. Early delivery, usually by induction of labour, should be undertaken by 38 weeks of gestation and may reduce perinatal mortality.

Acute fatty liver of pregnancy

Acute fatty liver of pregnancy is a rare condition and may be a variant of pre-eclampsia. It is a serious condition with a high maternal and fetal mortality of 15% and 25%, respectively. Early studies reported maternal mortality rates· of 80–90%. The condition usually presents in the third trimester with symptoms of nausea, malaise and vomiting; abdominal pain may subsequently develop. The features of pre-eclampsia (protein-uria and hypertension) are often present and the condition has to be differentiated from HELLP syndrome (see Chapter 6). Liver function tests are abnormal, with raised transaminases and alkaline phosphatase. In contrast to HELLP syndrome, acute fatty liver of pregnancy is associated with a marked hypoglycaemia and hyperuricaemia. Fulminant hepatic failure with encephalopathy, disseminated intravascular coagulation and renal failure may develop.

Liver histology shows microvesicular fatty infiltration of hepatocytes, especially in the central zone. However, liver biopsy is often omitted since it can be hazardous, especially in the presence of coagulopathy. The management of acute fatty liver of pregnancy is correction of any coagulopathy and hypoglycaemia and prompt delivery. These women may deteriorate rapidly and their management should involve a multidisciplinary team approach.

(X) OBESITY

Obesity, an increasing problem in Western society, has significant implications for pregnancy. There is a variety of definitions of obesity:

- specific weights of 80 kg or 90 kg body weight
- over 50% of ideal weight for height
- body mass index (BMI): weight (kg)/height (m)^2.

BMI is considered to be the best guide as it provides a measure of body fat content and allows standardisation for research (Table 7.14).

Table 7.14 Classification of weight by body mass index (BMI)	
Category	BMI
Low	<19.8
Medium	19.8–26
High	27–29
Obese	>29

The effect of obesity on pregnancy

Obese women are at greater risk of pregnancy complications and should be regarded as 'high-risk' (Table 7.15). Women with central (abdominal) obesity may have some difficulty conceiving. This reflects problems such as polycystic ovary syndrome and peripheral conversion of oestrogens to androgens, which disturbs ovarian function leading to oligomenorrhoea. Weight reduction often precipitates a normal menstrual cycle. A reduction in insulin resistance with insulin sensitising agents, such as metformin, may also restore ovulation, thus implicating insulin resistance in the disturbance of ovulation.

Miscarriage rates increase by around one-third when BMI is in excess of 25. The risk of hypertension and pre-eclampsia is increased. It is critical to use a wide blood-pressure cuff in order to avoid a false high blood

Table 7.15 Maternal complications in pregnancy associated with obesity
• Infertility
• Miscarriage
• Chronic hypertension and pre-eclampsia
• Gestational diabetes mellitus
• Thromboembolic disease
• Psychosocial problems
• Increased caesarean section rate
• Increased wound infection and dehiscence
• Respiratory impairment
• Urinary tract infections
• Dysfunctional labour

pressure reading. In women over 90 kg at term (approximately 95th centile for weight), the risk of chronic hypertension is of the order of four times that of the non-obese individual. These women are insulin resistant and because of this have an increased frequency of gestational diabetes and hypertriglyceridaemia. There is an increased risk of thromboembolic disease, which reflects not only their obesity but also their tendency to develop other complications of pregnancy, their associated immobility and the increased incidence of operative delivery. While this risk may be maximal postpartum, these women are still at high risk of antenatal thromboembolic problems. Antenatal thromboprophylaxis should be considered, particularly if additional risk factors are present.

Obese women have a high caesarean section rate even after adjusting for confounding variables such as gestational diabetes, hypertension and fetal macrosomia. Abdominal wound infections and dehiscence are more common. Episiotomy problems, particularly infection, are common and urinary tract infections occur more frequently. Morbidly obese women often have significant respiratory impairment, which has been associated with hypoxia. Thus, when operative delivery is required it is usually preferable for this to be carried out under regional block, although this might be technically difficult.

The fetus may also have problems (Table 7.16). There is a significant increase in neural tube defects for women with a prepregnancy BMI over 29, after adjusting for age, education, smoking status, alcohol use, chronic illness and vitamin use (Figure 7.3). Fetal macrosomia is more common and is independent of gestational diabetes. The prepregnancy weight has the strongest effect on birth weight and is more important than weight gain. Higher birth weights appear to reflect increased deposition of subcutaneous fat rather than an increase in linear growth. These infants tend to be obese in the first year of life. Shoulder dystocia is more common and is related to the macrosomia. Fetal distress is more common.

Table 7.16 Fetal and infant problems associated with obesity

- Increased risk of neural tube defect
- Fetal macrosomia
- Shoulder dystocia
- Fetal distress
- Neonatal and infant obesity

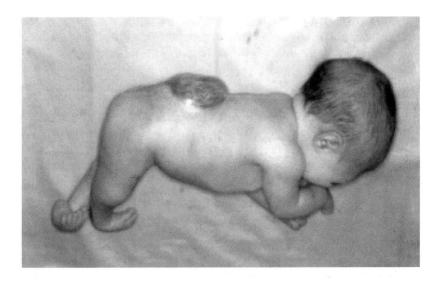

Figure 7.3 Obese women (body mass index >29) have a significant increase in the incidence of fetal neural-tube defects

Management of obesity in pregnancy

PREPREGNANCY

In prepregnancy counselling, it is vital to stress the importance of weight loss prior to conception. The aim of this is to reduce the BMI as close to normal as possible. This is important for pregnancy complications and fertility. Realistic and achievable targets should be set and dieticians and specialists in human nutrition can greatly facilitate this. The woman must also be counselled about the specific risks (Tables 7.15 and 7.16), as these may have significant consequences for her in terms of morbidity and management of the pregnancy. The problems associated with delivery should be discussed. In view of the increase in risk of neural tube defect these women should start folic acid supplements prior to conception, although there are no data with regard to the effectiveness of these supplements in patients who are obese.

ANTENATAL MANAGEMENT

At the first visit, it is important to discuss the risks and formulate a management plan. The woman should be screened for gestational diabetes, although there are no data to guide the timing and frequency of such screening. A pragmatic approach would be to screen early in the pregnancy, perhaps shortly after booking, around mid-pregnancy and perhaps late in the second or early in the third trimester. Consideration of risk factors for thrombosis must be borne in mind. Obesity on its own usually merits thromboprophylaxis but the timing of this will often depend on additional complications. For example, many women with morbid obesity have marked restriction in their mobility during pregnancy due to a combination of their size and discomfort associated with their weight, while separation of the symphysis may severely restrict mobility. When the obese patient is fully mobile and has no other risk factors, it is the practice at Glasgow Royal Infirmary not to employ pharmacological thromboprophylaxis. However, where mobility is significantly reduced, which often occurs in the third trimester, or other risk factors are present (see Section viii, Table 7.23), pharmacological thromboprophylaxis using low molecular weight heparin is employed. A suitable regimen would be 40 mg enoxaparin or 5000 units dalteparin sodium daily. For the very obese woman it may be of value to use twice daily dosing with low molecular weight heparin (e.g. enoxaparin 40 mg or dalteparin 5000 units) or a higher once-daily dose. The choice of dose is empirical. Thromboembolic deterrent stockings can be considered, although it is usually impossible to obtain stockings that fit correctly.

Weight must be monitored throughout the pregnancy. There is no need for obese women to gain the amount of weight normally associated with or recommended for pregnancy. Thus, static or modest weight loss is not associated with fetal problems. Modest weight loss or weight containment can be achieved by carbohydrate restriction without precipitating ketonuria.

An accurate measure of gestational age is required. It is often difficult to image the fetus and transvaginal scanning is useful in the first trimester. In later pregnancy it may be difficult to image fetal anatomy and this is important in view of the increased risk of neural tube defect. Imaging can usually be achieved when the BMI is lower than 35 but above this imaging may be unsatisfactory. Fetal growth must be monitored by ultrasound scanning, as abdominal examination is useless in the assessment of fetal growth, lie and presentation. In the third trimester, fortnightly scanning is recommended.

INTRAPARTUM MANAGEMENT

A short labour and an uncomplicated spontaneous vaginal delivery are the ideal, but the risk of dysfunctional labour and fetal problems reduce the likelihood of this. Should problems such as dysfunctional labour or fetal distress occur, the obstetrician would then be faced with the situation of an emergency caesarean section, which, in a morbidly obese patient, is extremely hazardous from anaesthetic and obstetric viewpoints. Emergency caesarean sections have an increased risk of wound complications and thromboembolism. Thus, elective caesarean section is often the best, or least hazardous, mode of delivery.

Caesarean section should be discussed with the anaesthetist regarding the timing of delivery and type of anaesthesia. A low transverse incision is usually best. The surgeon must decide whether to go under the panniculus or through it. If the latter approach is required, the surgeon must take care not to cut through the panniculus, emerging on its inferior surface rather than in the abdomen. With the former approach an extra assistant is usually required to hold up the panniculus. Access can be difficult due to the depth of the wound. Intra-abdominal and abdominal wall drains should be used, because of the increased risk of haematoma. Interrupted sutures or staples allow easy release and evacuation of any haematoma or serous collection.

If labour is planned induction is common, as there is a greater tendency for the woman to pass the expected date of delivery, as well as develop other complications. It is useful to have venous access established at an early stage. The anaesthetists must be aware of the woman's progress in labour. Shoulder dystocia should be anticipated.

POSTPARTUM MANAGEMENT

In the postpartum period it is important to provide thromboprophylaxis. Pragmatic management at the Glasgow Royal Infirmary is to provide a minimum of six weeks' thromboprophylaxis with subcutaneous injections of low molecular weight heparin (enoxaparin 40 mg/day or dalteparin 5000 units/day) or low molecular weight heparin followed by warfarin, aiming for a therapeutic international normalised ratio (INR) of 2–2.5 by the end of the first postpartum week. It is safe to breastfeed both on heparin and warfarin. Weight loss should be encouraged, although this should be avoided while breastfeeding is being established. Once feeding is established, patients can lose up to 2 kg/month without influencing their milk production, which contrasts with the higher calorific intake required for lactating women of normal weight.

(XI) RENAL DISEASE

Physiological changes in renal function with pregnancy

During pregnancy there is dilatation of the urinary collecting system. These changes are more marked on the right-hand side where the dilatation seen in the ureter can mimic obstructive uropathy. Blood flow to the kidneys increases by 60–80% in the first trimester and declines slightly in the third trimester. Glomerular filtration rate and creatinine clearance increases by 50% and is associated with a reduction in serum creatinine and urea concentrations. Renal protein excretion increases during pregnancy. Up to 300 mg of total protein may be excreted in the urine of healthy women in 24 hours. There is a degree of water and sodium retention and the majority of women experience some oedema.

Chronic renal disease

EFFECT OF CHRONIC RENAL DISEASE ON PREGNANCY

The problems for the mother and the risk to the fetus are dependent on the degree of renal compromise. Women with mild renal impairment (serum creatinine less than 125 μmol/l) tend to have a good outcome, whereas those with moderate (creatinine 125–275 μmol/l) to severe (creatinine over 275 μmol/l) impairment have a high incidence of problems. The mother will be at risk of pre-eclampsia, which can be difficult to identify in women with pre-existing proteinuria and hypertension. Blood pressure and renal function must be monitored carefully and hypertension treated. There is an association with intrauterine growth restriction and, thus, fetal growth and well-being should be monitored regularly. Preterm labour and iatrogenic preterm delivery in maternal or fetal interest is common. A significant decline in renal function often triggers preterm delivery. When proteinuria worsens but blood pressure remains normal or easily controlled and overall renal function stable or minimally affected, the pregnancy can be allowed to continue with suitable monitoring.

EFFECT OF PREGNANCY ON CHRONIC RENAL DISEASE

In connective tissue disorders (see Section VI) such as scleroderma, SLE and polyarteritis nodosa, renal function may deteriorate rapidly. Pregnancy may be best avoided in these conditions. Women with moderate to severe renal dysfunction must be warned of the risk of deterioration in their renal function. Reversible causes of reduction in renal function should also be considered such as urinary tract infection.

Women on dialysis and with transplant

Women on long-term haemodialysis or chronic ambulatory peritoneal dialysis have impaired fertility and conception is not common. When it does occur there is a high rate of miscarriage. The prospects of success are poor and the risk to the mother is great. Thus, therapeutic termination may be offered. There is a high risk of pre-eclampsia, growth restriction, severe hypertension and volume overload.

Following renal transplantation, normal endocrine function is often restored rapidly. It is not uncommon for women to become pregnant soon after renal transplantation. Despite the transplant, there is a high incidence of miscarriage and a high risk of pregnancy complications such as intrauterine growth restriction or pre-eclampsia. If transplant recipients do wish to become pregnant they should ideally wait two years after the transplantation to allow graft function to stabilise. Pregnancy does not appear to alter the long-term prognosis for the mother.

MANAGEMENT

Prepregnancy counselling is important in order to discuss the implications of pregnancy, which depend on the severity of renal compromise, the underlying disease and the presence of hypertension. Patients on dialysis or with transplants must be warned of the very high risk of pregnancy-related problems. Counsellors should take into account the patient's overall prognosis. Many patients with severe renal compromise and underlying disorders may themselves have a limited prognosis with regard to their health and their life. They must be aware that, should severe problems occur, termination of pregnancy may be required.

If pregnancy occurs, monitoring of the maternal and fetal condition must be carried out regularly. Collaboration between renal physicians and an obstetrician with a special interest in medical disorders or renal problems in pregnancy is optimal. Renal function should be assessed regularly with creatinine clearance, quantitative proteinuria and serum biochemistry. Anaemia associated with renal compromise will require treatment with haematinics and may require transfusion or recombinant erythropoietin.

Fetal growth and umbilical artery Doppler waveform analysis should be monitored from the second half of pregnancy, together with biophysical monitoring, particularly where intrauterine growth restriction occurs. Pre-eclampsia is difficult to diagnose in these women since their biochemistry may be abnormal and proteinuria and hypertension already present. Optimum control of blood pressure must occur. Patient and clinicians must be aware of the risk of preterm labour. Following delivery renal function can deteriorate. It is important to monitor renal function and control of blood pressure following delivery. Blood pressure control can be achieved with adrenoceptor antagonists, calcium channel blockers and methyldopa.

Low-dose aspirin (75 mg daily) from the end of the first trimester should be considered to prevent intrauterine growth restriction and pre-eclampsia, particularly in patients with an underlying connective tissue problem such as SLE. The decision to use aspirin in patients with moderate to severe renal problems should involve the nephrologist, as chronic inhibition of prostaglandin synthesis in the kidneys may occur.

(XII) NEUROLOGICAL DISEASE

Epilepsy in pregnancy

Epilepsy affects about 0.5% of women of childbearing age and is common in obstetric practice. These women have particular problems which are best addressed before conception, including contraception and prepregnancy counselling, as well as particular problems throughout pregnancy. Most women with epilepsy have no underlying cause for their seizures (idiopathic epilepsy). Epilepsy presenting for the first time in pregnancy is uncommon and should be differentiated from eclampsia, which is usually associated with hypertension and/or proteinuria. Any patient having such a seizure should have a full neurological assessment and objective investigations to exclude intracerebral tumours, arteriovenous malformations and cerebral venous thrombosis. These women have a higher incidence of underlying structural lesions than do nonpregnant patients presenting with a first seizure.

EFFECT OF EPILEPSY AND ANTICONVULSANTS ON PREGNANCY

Epilepsy and anticonvulsants have several effects on pregnancy (Table 7.17). Women with epilepsy tend to be less fertile than normal; in men, anticonvulsant medication may alter sperm motility and reduce circulating testosterone concentrations. There is an increased incidence of pregnancy complications including hyperemesis, anaemia, vaginal bleeding and intrauterine growth restriction. The anaemia may be related to folic acid antagonism by anticonvulsant drugs but the other complications are poorly understood.

There is a risk of the child itself developing epilepsy (Table 7.18). The effect of convulsions on fetal well-being depends upon the duration of

Table 7.17 Effects of epilepsy and anticonvulsants on pregnancy

- Pregnancy complications increased

  Hyperemesis

  Anaemia

  Vaginal bleeding

  Fetus small for dates
- Vitamin K and folic acid antagonism
- Fetal abnormality
- Haemorrhagic disease of the newborn
- Increased risk of epilepsy in offspring with maternal age of onset at under 18 years or seizures in pregnancy
- Neurodevelopmental problems and learning difficulties

Table 7.18 Risks of child of epileptic mother developing epilepsy

Epilepsy	Risk (%)
Either parent	4
Sibling	10
Both parents	15–20

the seizure. Fetal bradycardias have been reported during and following single grand mal seizures, but longer-term neurological impairment has not been consistently reported. In contrast, status epilepticus is harmful to both maternal and fetal health. Furthermore, children born of mothers with epilepsy may also suffer from neurodevelopmental problems and learning difficulties that may be related to exposure of the developing brain to anticonvulsants.

The main concern of women with epilepsy in pregnancy is an associated increase in fetal abnormalities (Table 7.19). The incidence of fetal abnormalities in the general population is about 3%. This risk is slightly increased (4%) in children whose parents have epilepsy but who are not taking anticonvulsant medication. The risk is further increased if the woman is taking anticonvulsants. The commonly used anticonvulsants (carbamazepine, phenobarbitone, phenytoin and sodium valproate) are teratogenic. The risk of fetal abnormality with any one drug is 6–7% and the risk increases with the number of drugs taken. The common fetal

Table 7.19 Fetal abnormalities associated with epilepsy	
Degree	*Abnormality*
Major	Neural tube defect
	Cardiac defect
	Cleft lip and palate
Minor	Club foot
	Hypospadias
Dysmorphic feature	Hypertelorism
	Long philtrum
	Low-set ears
	Wide mouth
	Irregular teeth
	Hypoplasia of distal phalanges and nails

abnormalities encountered are cleft lip and palate (Figure 7.4), cardiac defects and neural tube defects. Minor abnormalities include club foot and hypospadias. Furthermore, dysmorphic features can be seen such as hypoplasia of distal phalanges and nails, hypertelorism, low-set ears, long philtrum, irregular teeth and a wide mouth. Phenytoin has been associated with minor abnormalities in up to 30% of infants and with major defects in 5%. The incidence of orofacial clefts and congenital heart defects with phenytoin is about 1.5–2%. The most important abnormalities associated with sodium valproate ingestion are neural tube defects (1.5%) and congenital heart defects. Carbamazepine is also associated with an increased risk of neural tube defect (0.5%). The effects of the newer anticonvulsants (vigabatrin, lamotrigine and gabapentin) remain to be determined. While evidence suggests that the teratogenic risks of carbamazepine are less than the other drugs, if a woman is well controlled on other drugs, there is no indication to alter her medication. Clonazepam (a benzodiazepine) is not teratogenic.

The hepatic enzyme-inducing agents (primidone, phenobarbitone, phenytoin and carbamazepine) antagonise vitamin K, thereby reducing the vitamin K-dependent clotting factors. This will, in turn, expose the neonate to an increased risk of haemorrhagic disease of the newborn. This may be dealt with by prescribing vitamin K supplements to the mother in late pregnancy and also providing the neonate with vitamin K at the time of delivery. There is no contraindication to women breast-feeding while on anticonvulsants.

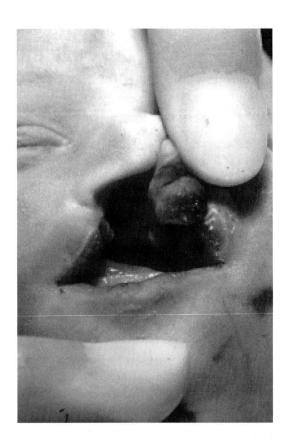

Figure 7.4 Common fetal abnormalities associated with anticonvulsant therapy include cleft lip and palate (shown here), cardiac defects and neural-tube defects

Phenobarbitone may result in the baby being sedated and lead to subsequent difficulties with feeding. Neonatal hepatic immaturity results in a considerable prolongation of the half-life of phenobarbitone. If the baby is sedated with the breast milk, breastfeeding should occur before the woman takes her anticonvulsant medication. Alternatively, these babies may experience jitteriness on withdrawal if they are not breastfed.

EFFECT OF PREGNANCY ON EPILEPSY AND ANTICONVULSANTS

Pregnancy has an effect on epilepsy and anticonvulsant treatment. Up to one-quarter of women show an increase in seizure frequency, up to one-quarter show a decline and up to one-half remain unchanged. The change in frequency is unpredictable and is not influenced by the type of seizure, anticonvulsant medication or the woman's age. Patients with poorly controlled epilepsy are more likely to experience an increase in their seizure frequency. These changes may be related to the hormonal and metabolic alterations of pregnancy; sleep deprivation, stress, hyperventilation and exhaustion, particularly in labour and, in addition, may relate to non-compliance (Table 7.20). Non-compliance is relatively common, as women are aware of the potential problems of anticonvulsant drugs with regard to fetal abnormalities. Unfortunately, most women discontinue therapy after the window for teratogenesis has passed.

Most anticonvulsant drugs show a fall in total levels during pregnancy due to changes in plasma protein binding and drug clearance yet most patients see no increase in seizure frequency. This is because free drug levels change much less than the total drug level. This has implications for monitoring therapy during pregnancy. For example, for a decline in total phenytoin levels of around 56%, the free drug level will decline by just over 30%. With sodium valproate, the total drug levels may fall by 39% but the free drug levels increase by 25%. Thus, while drug levels may confirm compliance, their assessment does not provide a reliable guide on which to base dose adjustments. In general terms, the dose should be adjusted

- if there is an increase in seizure frequency, provided compliance is confirmed
- if there are adverse effects
- if there are gross changes in drug levels (excluding non-compliance) that would be likely to lead to the patient being at high risk of having a seizure.

Management of epilepsy

PREPREGNANCY COUNSELLING

Prepregnancy counselling by general practitioners, obstetricians and physicians, should be provided to all women with epilepsy of childbearing age. They should be advised of the increased risk of abnormalities

Table 7.20 Reasons for an increase in seizure frequency during pregnancy
• Poor compliance
• Nausea and vomiting decrease drug levels
• Increased volume of distribution and drug clearance
• Fatigue: impaired sleep towards term
• Impaired absorption of anticonvulsant medication during labour
• Labour: hyperventilation, failure to take medication, vomiting, lack of sleep

and dysmorphic features but it should be emphasised that the majority of babies born to mothers with epilepsy are normal. Preconceptual folic acid supplements should be commenced. The recommended dose is 5 mg/day for at least 12 weeks prior to conception and this dose should be continued throughout pregnancy to avoid folate-deficiency anaemia. The management of pregnancy should be discussed. Prenatal screening and diagnosis using serum testing and detailed ultrasound scanning to detect major fetal abnormalities must be offered. The woman should be informed that prolonged grand mal convulsions during pregnancy carry serious risks for both mother and fetus. Anticonvulsants should be continued to avoid this and her anticonvulsant therapy should be reviewed. The aim is to achieve good seizure control on monotherapy, if possible. Women who have been seizure-free for many years may consider discontinuing anticonvulsant medication. However, if drug treatment is adjusted or withdrawn the clinician must counsel adequately regarding possible implications to the patient's life in the event of a seizure, including loss of her driving licence and implications for her job.

ANTENATAL MANAGEMENT

Ideally, women with epilepsy should be managed in a consultant unit with a team with a special interest in such conditions. Seizure control and drugs should be carefully noted and also folic acid prescribed. Fetal abnormality screening should be carried out (Figure 7.5). Blood levels can be monitored to check compliance. Drugs should not be altered without expert advice simply on the basis of drug levels. Vitamin K should be commenced in a dose of 20 mg orally from 36 weeks of gestation or earlier if preterm delivery is anticipated and vitamin K given intra-muscularly to the baby at birth.

INTRAPARTUM MANAGEMENT

Women with epilepsy should be managed in a consultant unit and obviously should avoid birthing techniques such as the use of the birthing pool. Anticonvulsant agents should be continued through labour and ideally doses should not be missed as there is likely to be an increase in stress, hyperventilation and sleep deprivation during the course of labour, which may trigger seizures.

POSTNATAL MANAGEMENT

Postpartum, women should be encouraged to breastfeed. If drugs have been increased in dose during pregnancy this should be reduced gradually

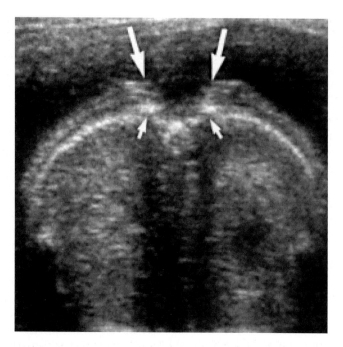

Figure 7.5 Ultrasound scan showing a neural tube defect; in view of the increased risk of such defects associated with anticonvulsant therapy in pregnancy, prenatal screening and diagnosis should be offered routinely to women who have had this therapy

to the prepregnancy level following delivery. The baby should be carefully examined for fetal abnormalities. Reassurance and care should be given with regard to infant care. The infant should be dressed on a changing mat on the floor and the mother should not bathe the infant unaccompanied. She may find it reassuring to attach a cord from her wrist to the pram when walking outdoors. Contraception should be discussed.

CONTRACEPTION

The effectiveness of hormonal contraception is reduced in women on anticonvulsants which are hepatic enzyme-inducing (carbamazepine, phenytoin, primidone and phenobarbitone). Sodium valproate, vigabatrin, lamotrigine, gabapentin and the benzodiazepines do not have this effect. If a combined oestrogen-containing oral contraceptive pill is used this should contain at least 50 μg of oestradiol per day (Table 7.21). The blood progesterone concentration can be measured on day 21 to ensure that ovulation is inhibited. Some women will need up to 100 μg of

Table 7.21 Hormonal contraception for women taking enzyme inducing anticonvulsants

Contraceptive	Comments
Combined oral contraceptive pill	50 μg ethinyl oestradiol pill (or 2 × 25 μg ethinyl oestradiol pills) should be used initially with a reduced pill-free interval
Progesterone-only pill	Should only be used if no other acceptable method
	Doubling of the daily dose may be effective
Parenteral-progestogen	Reduce dosing interval from 12 weeks to 10 weeks

oestradiol per day to inhibit ovulation. Contraceptive cover can be enhanced by reducing the pill-free interval to four days and by using four packs of pills consecutively. This may have the additional benefit of preventing hormonally triggered seizures at the time of menstruation. Liver enzyme-inducing drugs also increase the metabolism of progestogens and women should take at least double the usual dose. Alternatively, non-hormonal methods should be used.

Multiple sclerosis

Multiple sclerosis affects up to 0.1% of the population in the UK and tends to present during the childbearing years. Its aetiology is unknown and it is characterised by multiple areas of demyelination within the brain and spinal cord. It tends to be a relapsing and remitting condition with lesions occurring in different parts of the central nervous system at different times. Alternatively, it can be a chronic progressive disorder.

Multiple sclerosis is unlikely to present for the first time during pregnancy and is also less likely to relapse during pregnancy. Those women with bladder involvement may be prone to recurrent urinary tract infections and urine should be sent for bacteriological investigation at each antenatal visit. Consideration should be given to prophylactic antibiotics. Almost half of women with multiple sclerosis will experience an exacerbation in the six months post-delivery but there are no long-term detrimental effects of pregnancy or breastfeeding on the course of the disease. Similarly, multiple sclerosis tends to have no effect on the course of the pregnancy.

Myasthenia gravis

Myasthenia gravis is characterised by weakness and fatiguability of proximal limb, ocular and bulbar muscles. The aetiology is unknown, although thymic hyperplasia is found in 70% of these patients and a thymic tumour in 10%. IgG antibodies to the nicotinic acetylcholine receptor are found which interfere with neurotransmission at the post-synaptic membrane. The prevalence is about 4/100 000 and it is twice as common in women as in men. Most patients with myasthenia gravis are treated with long-acting anticholinesterases.

In about one-third of women, there is no change in disease activity during pregnancy, in one-third remissions occur and in the other third the disease is exacerbated. Disease activity may deteriorate during pregnancy because of alterations in the ingestion, absorption, volume of distribution and clearance of drug treatment. The long-acting anticholinesterases (pyridostigmine bromide) are not known to be teratogenic. A number of drugs commonly used in pregnancy are contraindicated in the disease (Table 7.22).

The condition has no effect on the myometrial smooth muscle and consequently no effect upon the first stage of labour. Maternal effort in the expulsive phase of the second stage may be compromised and an instrumental delivery may be required. Myasthenia gravis is associated with preterm delivery and intrauterine growth restriction. The IgG antibodies implicated in myasthenia gravis can cross the placenta and up to 20% of neonates may experience transient neonatal myasthenia gravis, which usually resolves within two months.

Table 7.22 Drug interactions in myasthenia gravis	
Drug	*Comment*
Ether	
Halothane	
Ester-type local anaesthetics	If concurrent treatment with anticholinesterases
Non-depolarising muscle relaxants	Increased sensitivity
Aminoglycoside antibiotics and clindamycin	Antagonise effects of anticholinesterases
Betasympathomimetics	Exacerbate the disease
Magnesium sulphate	May precipitate a crisis
Antimalarials	Exacerbate the disease

(XIII) HAEMOSTASIS AND THROMBOSIS

Physiological changes in pregnancy

Changes within the maternal circulation during pregnancy and the puerperium result in an increased thrombotic potential. Changes in coagulation factors during pregnancy favour thrombosis. There are significant increases in factors I, VII, VIII, IX, X, XII, von Willebrand factor antigen and ristocetin co-factor activity, the functional assessment of von Willebrand factor. There is a reduction in the endogenous anticoagulant protein S, while the activated protein C sensitivity ratio falls. Fibrinolytic activity is impaired during pregnancy, due to placentally derived plasminogen activator inhibitor type II and an increase in plasminogen activator type I. Venous blood flow is substantially altered during pregnancy and a marked reduction in blood flow velocity occurs by the early part of the second trimester, reaching a nadir at 34 weeks to term and taking six weeks to return to normal values postnatally. This decrease in flow is more marked in the left common femoral vein than in the right. Consistent with this, around 85% of deep venous thromboses (DVT) that occur in pregnancy arise in the left leg compared with 55% outwith pregnancy. Trauma to the pelvic veins may occur during normal vaginal delivery and particularly so during abdominal or instrumental delivery.

Thromboembolic disease in pregnancy

Pulmonary thromboembolism remains the main cause of maternal death in the UK. Many thromboses go unnoticed until the fatal event occurs. The diagnosis of DVT is important since pulmonary thromboembolism will arise in 16% of patients with DVT left untreated, resulting in a 13% mortality rate. With early anticoagulant therapy, the mortality rate of DVT is reduced to 0.7%. The incidence of antenatal DVT in Scotland is 0.615 per 1000 maternities in women under the age of 35 years and 1.216 per 1000 maternities in women over the age of 35 years. The incidence of pulmonary thromboembolism is 0.108 per 1000 maternities in those under 35 years and 0.405 per 1000 maternities in those over 35 years. Delivery by caesarean section and, in particular, emergency caesarean section, is associated with an increased risk of venous thromboembolism. The risk factors for venous thromboembolism in pregnancy are summarised in Table 7.23.

THROMBOPHILIA

The body has natural anticoagulant systems. These take the form of the antithrombin system and activated protein C/protein S systems.

Table 7.23 Risk factors for venous thrombosis in pregnancy

- Age over 35 years
- Immobility
- Obesity
- Operative delivery
- Pre-eclampsia
- Parity greater than four
- Surgical procedure in pregnancy or puerperium, e.g., postpartum sterilisation
- Previous deep vein thrombosis
- Thrombophilia
  Congenital
      antithrombin deficiency
      protein C deficiency
      protein S deficiency
      factor V Leiden
      prothrombin gene variant
  Acquired
      lupus anticoagulant
      anticardiolipin antibodies
- Excessive blood loss
- Paraplegia
- Sickle cell disease
- Inflammatory disorders and infection, e.g., inflammatory bowel disease and urinary tract infection
- Dehydration

Antithrombin inhibits many activated coagulation factors such as factor Xa and IIa. Its action is enhanced by binding with heparin and this is the mechanism by which heparin exerts its anticoagulant effect. When the coagulation system is activated, thrombin binds to thrombomodulin on the endothelial cell surface. This in turn activates protein C which, along with its co-factor, protein S, will inhibit factor VIIIa and factor Va by proteolytic cleavage. Deficiency of antithrombin, protein C or protein S will result in increased risk of thrombosis.

Many DVTs occurring in young women during the course of pregnancy are the first manifestation of underlying thrombophilic problems. The most common problem being factor V Leiden which has a gene frequency of 3–10% in Western populations. Factor V Leiden is an abnormal form of factor V. It has normal coagulation function but is resistant to breakdown by activated protein C, resulting in an increase in thrombotic risk. Investigations of patients with a DVT in pregnancy may find factor V Leiden in over 20% of cases. It is also associated with thrombotic problems on the oral contraceptive pill.

Deficiencies of the endogenous anticoagulants antithrombin, protein C and protein S are much less common than factor V Leiden and taken together they will be found in around only 5% of women with a DVT in pregnancy. Antithrombin deficiency carries the highest risk of venous thrombosis in pregnancy. Thrombosis, which occurs in association with protein C and protein S deficiency, will usually occur postpartum. More recently, a variant has been found in a prothrombin gene with those being heterozygous having higher levels of prothrombin and an enhanced risk of thrombosis.

Any patient presenting with thromboembolism in pregnancy should be screened for underlying congenital or acquired thrombophilia. Screening may have to be delayed until after anticoagulant therapy is completed as anticoagulants will interfere with some of the tests used for the assessment of these abnormalities. Any patient with a past history or significant family history of thrombosis should also be screened.

Clinical features and diagnosis of venous thromboembolism

DEEP VENOUS THROMBOSIS

Clinical diagnosis of DVT is unreliable. Less than half of all cases of DVT involving proximal veins are identified. In many maternal deaths from pulmonary thromboembolism, DVT is found for the first time at autopsy. Most of the symptoms and signs of DVT occur as a result of venous outflow obstruction and inflammation of the venous wall and surrounding tissues. None is specific to DVT. The clinical diagnosis of DVT is further hampered during pregnancy as leg swelling and discomfort occur commonly in normal pregnancy. Thus, the role of clinical evaluation is to identify the patient at risk. Objective testing should be employed to confirm or refute the diagnosis. Duplex Doppler ultrasound, which is non-invasive with a high sensitivity and specificity, is the first-line investigation of choice (Figure 7.6). It is limited in its

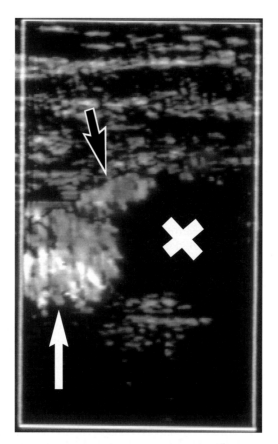

Figure 7.6 Doppler ultrasound scan showing blood flow in the femoral artery (closed arrow) and in a superficial vein (open arrow); there is no flow in the common femoral vein (cross), indicating a femoral-vein thrombosis

ability to delineate major thrombosis in the iliac vessels above the level of the inguinal ligament and cannot easily provide comprehensive visualisation of all calf veins. Nonetheless, it would be unusual for a large iliac vein thrombosis not to produce either extension to the femoral vein or alteration in the flow, which would be apparent on ultrasound examination. If there is significant doubt, X-ray venography with shielding of the abdomen should be performed. Most DVTs in pregnancy arise on the left and in contrast to the non-pregnancy situation are predominantly ileofemoral rather than popliteofemoral. This is important, as ileofemoral thrombi are more likely to break off and become pulmonary thromboembolic.

PULMONARY THROMBOEMBOLISM

The clinical diagnosis of pulmonary thromboembolism is unreliable. Autopsy findings indicate that no more than one-third of emboli are diagnosed clinically.

THE MOST COMMON CLINICAL FEATURES OF PATIENTS WITH OBJECTIVELY CONFIRMED ACUTE PULMONARY THROMBOEMBOLISM

- Dyspnoea
- Tachypnoea
- Pleuritic chest pain
- Hypotension
- Tachycardia
- Cough
- Haemoptysis
- Leg pain

In the nonpregnant patient, the predictive value of any single feature in diagnosing or excluding pulmonary thromboembolism is less than 80%. Despite the variety of symptoms associated with pulmonary thromboembolism, patients tend to present in one of three ways:

- circulatory collapse with hypotension and/or loss of consciousness, with or without central chest tightness
- pulmonary haemorrhage with pleuritic chest pain and/or haemoptysis
- isolated dyspnoea.

Of note, dyspnoea, tachypnoea and leg discomfort may be physiological during pregnancy, particularly in the third trimester when dyspnoea is most apparent at rest. Clinical examination of the patient with pulmonary thromboembolism may reveal a rapid respiratory rate but only a small proportion of patients have a demonstrable friction rub. Massive pulmonary thromboembolism will be associated with cyanosis, hypotension and an elevated jugular venous pressure.

The initial assessment of women in whom there is clinical suspicion of pulmonary thromboembolism should include chest X-ray, electrocardiography (ECG) and an evaluation of arterial blood gases. The chest X-ray may be normal and its value is in the exclusion of other conditions such as pneumothorax and pneumonia. Common radiological findings in pulmonary thromboembolism include focal infiltrate, segmental collapse, raised diaphragm (a normal feature of pregnancy) and pleural effusion; wedge-shaped infarction is a rare finding. The ECG may be normal except for a sinus tachycardia; abnormalities that may be present include S waves in lead I, Q waves in leads II and III and non-specific changes in the ST segment and/or T wave. Right axis deviation may be present with a large pulmonary thromboembolism. The normal pregnancy-related changes in the ECG may also make interpretation difficult. The arterial blood gases in pulmonary thromboembolism may reveal a reduced Pao_2 and a normal or low $Paco_2$, although normal Pao_2 and $Paco_2$ values may be found, particularly with smaller emboli. It should be noted that $Paco_2$ and HCO_3^- values are lower in normal pregnancy due to a chronic mild respiratory alkalosis. The risk of haemorrhage from the arterial puncture site in the presence of anticoagulation is significant, and pulse oximetry represents a less invasive method of determining oxygen saturation.

Once the patient is stabilised, specific investigations are required to confirm the diagnosis of pulmonary thromboembolism. The ventilation-perfusion scan (V/Q scan) remains the first-line test in the evaluation of suspected pulmonary thromboembolism in pregnancy. Since the ventilation phase rarely adds to the accuracy of the scan, the perfusion phase is normally performed first, particularly as young women do not commonly have chronic chest problems leading to matched ventilation-perfusion defects. Further, a normal perfusion scan, while not completely excluding pulmonary thromboembolism, means that any emboli present are unlikely to be clinically significant and the ventilation scan can be omitted, thereby limiting the radiation dose. Perfusion scanning is performed by the intravenous injection of technetium (Tc-99m)-labelled macro-aggregates of albumin or human albumin microspheres. To minimise the radiation to the fetus, the dose of Tc-99m for perfusion studies can be reduced from 111 Bq to 74 or 37 Bq, without compromising the quality of the scan. Ideally, ventilation scans are performed with krypton (Kr-81m) or Tc-99m DTPA (diethylenetriaminepentaacetic acid) aerosol, rather than xenon (^{133}Xe), since the former provide clearer multiview images, resulting in fewer intermediate scan reports. The combination of chest X-ray, V/Q scan and pulmonary angiography exposes the fetus to less than 5000 μGy (0.5 rad). Exposure to radiation of less than 50 000 μGy (5 rad) has not been associated with a significant risk of fetal injury. Doses in the range of 1–4 rad appear to carry a risk of oncogenicity of around 1/1000–1/2000 with risk relating particularly to exposure in early pregnancy and dose. In the puerperium, breastfeeding should be avoided for the following 15 hours. If the result is equivocal then ultrasound assessment of the leg veins is useful, as the diagnosis of DVT would lead to therapeutic anticoagulation whether or not a pulmonary embolism was present.

Pulmonary angiography is considered the gold standard in the diagnosis of pulmonary thromboembolism, although the technique is invasive and is virtually always unnecessary. It should be considered if cardiovascular collapse or hypotension is present and where other investigations have failed to give a firm diagnosis. The diagnosis of pulmonary thromboembolism is made at angiography by identifying the embolus as a constant intraluminal filling defect or by finding an abrupt cut-off of a pulmonary artery greater than 2.5 mm in diameter.

Helical computed tomography (Figure 7.7), magnetic resonance imaging (Figure 7.8) and measurement of plasma D-dimer have not been fully evaluated in pregnancy, but D-dimer is elevated in normal pregnancy and thus could only be used to exclude rather than confirm the diagnosis.

Management of DVT and pulmonary thromboembolism

Therapeutic doses of heparin are the mainstay of treatment of antenatal venous thromboembolism. Acute treatment with subcutaneous, unfractionated heparin administered twice daily may be used (15–20 000 iu twice daily). Alternatively, treatment may be initiated with an intravenous bolus of 5000 iu (or 75 iu/kg body weight) over five minutes followed by a continuous intravenous infusion for five to ten days. Thereafter, 12-hourly subcutaneous injections of heparin should be continued for the remainder of the pregnancy. Regardless of the route of

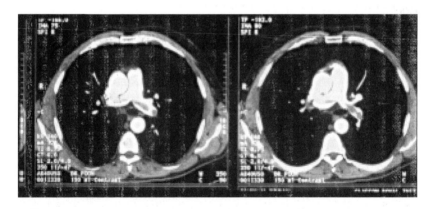

Figure 7.7 Helical computed tomography showing a saddle embolus at the bifurcation of the pulmonary artery; this technique employs large doses of radiation and its use in the diagnosis of pulmonary thromboembolism in pregnancy should be restricted to the postnatal period

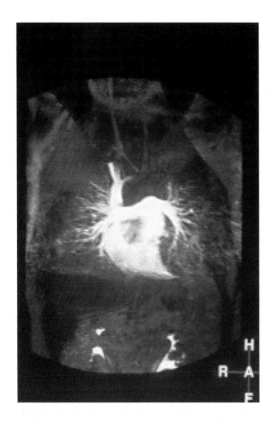

Figure 7.8 Magnetic resonance imaging may have a role in the diagnosis of pulmonary thromboembolism in pregnancy owing to its lack of ionising radiation

administration, treatment with unfractionated heparin should be monitored by the activated partial thromboplastin time (APTT) and the dose adjusted to maintain the mid-interval APTT at twice the control (range 1.5–2.5). There is an increasing realisation that APTT monitoring of unfractionated heparin is technically problematic, particularly in late pregnancy when an apparent heparin resistance occurs due to increased fibrinogen and factor VIII. This can lead to unnecessarily high doses of heparin being used, with subsequent haemorrhagic problems. When available, assessment of anti-Xa levels may be helpful in avoiding such inadvertent heparin overdose.

In nonpregnant patients, low molecular weight heparin (LMWH) is effective, safe and associated with fewer adverse effects than unfractionated heparin in the treatment of acute DVT and pulmonary thromboembolism. Initial treatment with LMWH is now the preferred management of DVT in nonpregnant subjects. The Glasgow Royal Infirmary now routinely uses the LMWH, enoxaparin, for immediate treatment of DVT and pulmonary thromboembolism in pregnancy. When antenatal venous thromboembolism is suspected, treatment with enoxaparin is commenced at a dose of 1 mg/kg subcutaneously, at 12-hourly intervals, based on early pregnancy weight, since LMWH does not cross the placenta. Enoxaparin is available in syringes of 40, 60, 80 and 100 mg, and the dose closest to the patient's weight is employed. Other LMWH, such as dalteparin or tinzaparin, could also be used at similar doses. Objective testing is undertaken and, if venous thromboembolism is confirmed, treatment is continued until delivery. Until further experience is obtained, it is recommended that treatment is monitored by measuring anti-Xa activity (target therapeutic range 0.4–1.0 unit/ml, three hours post-injection). The dose of enoxaparin is reduced to 40 mg 12-hourly during labour and therapeutic doses recommenced immediately following delivery. Initial experience suggests that a measurable anticoagulant effect (anti-Xa activity greater than 0.2 unit/ml) is maintained between drug administration. Further, there is no accumulation in the anticoagulant effect assessed by peak anti-Xa activity. Subcutaneous LMWH has advantages over APTT-monitored unfractionated heparin in the treatment of venous thromboembolism in pregnancy. The simplified therapeutic regimen for LMWH is convenient for patients and allows outpatient treatment. LMWH may be safe and effective for the treatment of venous thromboembolism in pregnancy and easier to initiate and administer than unfractionated heparin.

Heparin does not cross the placenta and there is no direct risk to the fetus, but it is not without hazard in pregnancy (Table 7.24). With long-term use, there is a risk of heparin-induced osteopenia, the risk of which relates poorly to dose and duration with problems being seen at doses as

Table 7.24 Anticoagulants in pregnancy: adverse effects and risks

Anticoagulant	Risk
Warfarin	Warfarin embryopathy
	mid-face hypoplasia
	frontal bossing
	stippled chondral calcification
	Fetal haemorrhage
	Maternal haemorrhage
Heparin	Allergy
	Osteoporosis
	Thrombocytopenia

low as 15 000 iu/day and after periods of treatment as short as seven weeks. It usually manifests clinically as vertebral crush fractures, which will occur in around 2% of women on long-term heparin therapy in pregnancy. Other complications are heparin-induced thrombocytopenia and heparin allergy. Heparin allergy normally manifests itself as raised erythematous plaques at heparin injection sites (Figure 7.9). Heparin allergy can sometimes be dealt with by switching between different heparins or from unfractionated to LMWH. Heparin-induced thrombocytopenia can be a serious problem in long-term heparin use occurring in 2–3% of patients on long-term heparin. In this situation, thrombotic problems can arise due to platelet activation. This is due to an antibody directed against a platelet/antibody complex. In view of this, platelet count should

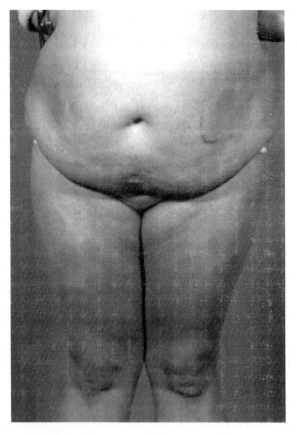

Figure 7.9 A patient with heparin allergy manifesting itself as raised erythematous plaques at the heparin injection sites (outer thighs and lower abdominal wall)

be checked regularly in all patients on heparin in pregnancy. LMWH carry substantially less risk of osteopenia, thrombocytopenia and allergy.

Warfarin should be avoided during pregnancy, since its use is associated with a characteristic embryopathy in the first trimester and adverse effects on the fetus throughout pregnancy (Table 7.24). Warfarin is associated with fetal and neonatal haemorrhage caused by markedly depressed production of vitamin K-dependent clotting factors in the fetus compounded by the trauma of delivery.

Anticoagulant treatment should be continued postpartum with either heparin or warfarin. Both heparin and warfarin are safe to use while breastfeeding. When oral anticoagulant therapy is initiated, it should be overlapped with heparin until the INR is greater than 2.0 on two consecutive days. Thereafter, the optimal target therapeutic range of the INR during anticoagulant therapy for a first episode of venous thromboembolism is 2.0–3.0. If there is a severe underlying thrombophilic problem, such as antiphospholipid antibody syndrome, the INR should be maintained between 3.0 and 3.5. Warfarin treatment should be continued for at least six weeks postpartum or until at least three months of anticoagulant therapy have been completed. Practice at Glasgow Royal Infirmary is to continue anticoagulant treatment for three months postnatally.

Inferior vena cava filters have been used successfully during pregnancy when, in contrast to nonpregnancy, suprarenal placement is recommended. The indications for their use are the same as in nonpregnant patients and include contraindication to anticoagulant therapy, serious complication of anticoagulation (e.g. heparin-induced thrombocytopenia) and recurrent pulmonary thromboembolism in patients with adequate anticoagulation. Thrombolysis with streptokinase or recombinant tissue plasminogen activator lyses pulmonary emboli more rapidly than conventional anticoagulation and should be considered in massive pulmonary thromboembolism during pregnancy. Antenatally, there is concern that this treatment may result in placental abruption. Further, thrombolysis should be avoided within six hours of delivery and in the early postpartum period because of the high risk of bleeding complications. Pulmonary embolectomy is rarely indicated and should only be considered in women with massive pulmonary thromboembolism who fail to respond to thrombolytic therapy over the first hour.

The patient with previous DVT

It is important in the antenatal assessment of any patient to enquire about her past medical history for any history of venous thromboembolic disease and any family history of such an event. If a patient has had a previous DVT, her risk will be increased during pregnancy. It is also important that she is screened for congenital or acquired thrombophilia. Ideally, these patients should be seen for prepregnancy assessment and counselling in order to ensure that they are aware of the risk of recurrence of venous thromboembolism in pregnancy and the problems of anticoagulants, both for the mother and the fetus. In patients with multiple previous venous thromboembolic problems it would be usual to initiate thromboprophylaxis at least four to six weeks in advance of the gestation at which the previous thrombosis occurred or, if not associated with pregnancy, in the middle of the second trimester. In any event, it would be usual to start treatment by 20 weeks of gestation. Additional risk factors would result in treatment being started earlier and even in the first trimester. The timing of such therapy will be particularly influenced by the presence of congenital or acquired thrombophilia, particularly with antithrombin deficiency. Such patients require specialist care from centres experienced in the management of thrombophilia in pregnancy.

In a patient with a single previous DVT, either within or outwith pregnancy, and no underlying thrombophilia, there is controversy as to whether antenatal prophylaxis is required in view of the risks of long-term heparin therapy and the relatively low risk of recurrence in the absence of thrombophilia. Each case should be judged on its merits. However, there is no doubt that postpartum thromboprophylaxis is essential. Thromboprophylaxis in pregnancy can be unfractionated heparin, LMWH, antiplatelet agents (low-dose aspirin) and thromboembolic deterrent stockings. Unfractionated heparin should be given in a dose of 10 000 iu twice daily after 20 weeks of gestation. LMWH, such as enoxaparin, should be administered in a dose of 40 mg once a day, or dalteparin 5000 iu once a day. LMWH has the advantage of once-daily administration and less risk of heparin-induced adverse effects (Table 7.25).

Indications for thromboprophylaxis in pregnancy

Thromboprophylaxis is not without its complications and, therefore, each woman should have her risk of venous thromboembolism assessed carefully and accurately. This may involve reviewing case notes to determine whether a previous diagnosis of venous thromboembolism was objectively diagnosed. Recommendations for thromboprophylaxis during pregnancy and the puerperium have been published by the Royal College of Obstetrics and Gynaecology, and a risk chart has been drawn up for women undergoing caesarean section (Table 7.26).

Inherited bleeding disorders in pregnancy

Haemorrhage during pregnancy may occur in association with specific complications of pregnancy (see Chapter 3) or it may be caused by an

7.25 Management of the patient with previous venous thromboembolism (VTE)

Thrombosis	Management
Previous deep vein thrombosis × 1	Exclude thrombophilia Discuss with the patient Antenatal vigilance Graduated elastic compression stockings ± low molecular weight heparin (or ? low-dose aspirin)
⩾VTE × 2; no thrombophilia	Low molecular weight heparin from early pregnancy
Symptomatic thrombophilia	Low molecular weight heparin from early pregnancy (higher dose or increased dose frequency required in high risk conditions, such as antithrombin deficiency and anticardiolipin antibodies)
Asymptomatic thrombophilia	Individual assessment Treatment depends on the thrombophilia Seek expert advice

inherited or acquired bleeding disorder. The most common inherited bleeding disorders are haemophilia A (factor VIII deficiency), haemophilia B (factor IX deficiency) and von Willebrand's disease (von Willebrand factor deficiency). Pregnant women with these disorders, or who are genetic carriers for them, and the female partners of men with these conditions should be managed at specialist clinics attended by obstetricians and haematologists.

HAEMOPHILIA A AND HAEMOPHILIA B

Haemophilia A and haemophilia B are X-linked recessive disorders with a prevalence in the UK of 90 per million and 20 per million, respectively. The majority of female carriers have no major bleeding problems, although the 10–20% of carriers who exhibit extreme Lyonisation are at risk of bleeding. Half of the male children of female carriers will inherit these disorders and are at risk of serious bleeding. The main bleeding problem in haemophilia is into joints and muscles, leading to debilitating arthritis. In these women, the bleeding time is normal since platelet function is normal. In haemophilia A, the activated partial thromboplastin time is prolonged, since factor VIII levels are reduced.

Table 7.26 Thromboembolic risk assessment in women undergoing caesarean section

Risk	Factors	Measures
Low	Elective caesarean section: uncomplicated pregnancy and no other risk factors	Early mobilisation and hydration
Moderate	Age over 35 years Obesity (>80 kg) High parity (para 4 or more) Gross varicose veins Current infection Pre-eclampsia Immobility prior to surgery (>4 days) Major current illness (e.g. heart or lung disease, cancer, inflammatory bowel disease) Emergency caesarean section in labour	Variety of prophylactic measures
High	A patient with 3 or more moderate risk factors from above Extended major pelvic or abdominal surgery (e.g. caesarean hysterectomy) Patients with a personal or family history of deep vein thrombosis, pulmonary thromboembolism, thrombophilia or paralysis of the limbs Patients with antiphospholipid antibody (cardiolipin antibody or lupus anticoagulant)	Low molecular weight heparin prophylaxis ± leg stockings

VON WILLEBRAND'S DISEASE

Von Willebrand's disease (vWD) is the most common clinically important inherited bleeding disorder affecting women, with a prevalence of up to 1%. The dysfunction is in platelet-endothelial interaction, which is mediated by von Willebrand's factor. These patients suffer mucosal bleeds: epistaxis, gastrointestinal bleeds and menorrhagia and have a prolonged bleeding time. Von Willebrand's factor may have a reduced functional activity assessed by reduced ristocetin co-factor activity and factor VIII activity, since it also carries factor VIII. Essentially, there are three types of vWD. Type I vWD is the most common type characterised by a reduction in all forms of von Willebrand's factor. It can have either an autosomal dominant or an autosomal recessive inheritance. In type II vWD, the highest molecular weight von Willebrand's factor multimers are lost and inheritance is usually autosomal dominant. Type II has sub-variants named IIA and IIB. Bleeding episodes in type II vWD tend to be more prolonged and more severe than in type I vWD. Type III vWD is clinically the most severe and is autosomal recessive in inheritance. These patients are usually homozygous and have a bleeding tendency that mimics moderately severe haemophilia A, with the added mucosal and subcutaneous bleeding characteristic of vWD.

In normal pregnancy, both factor VIII and von Willebrand's factor rise steadily, and most pregnant women with vWD also show an increase in these factors. In effect, most women with vWD do not have excessive bleeding during pregnancy and when bleeding does occur, it tends to happen postnatally and is associated with surgical delivery and perineal trauma. The concentrations of factor VIII and von Willebrand's factor fall rapidly after delivery. Further, women are more likely to have bleeding complications if they have types II and III vWD, rather than type I.

Management of pregnancies with haemorrhagic disorders

PRECONCEPTUAL COUNSELLING

Couples with a family history of heritable bleeding disorders should be informed of the genetic implications of their particular disorder and carriers should be identified before conception, to allow appropriate genetic counselling and recognition of those women at increased risk of haemorrhage. Women who may require treatment with blood products should be immunised against hepatitis A and hepatitis B. The availability of prenatal diagnosis, usually via chorionic villus sampling, should be discussed with carriers of the haemophilias.

ANTENATAL MANAGEMENT

Women with vWD and carriers of haemophilia A or B should have their antenatal care supervised jointly by an obstetrician with an interest in medical disorders and a haematologist. Coagulation factor activity and, if appropriate, levels of von Willebrand's factor antigen and ristocetin co-factor activity, should be determined at least every eight weeks. With vWD it is worth measuring bleeding time in late pregnancy. Assessment in the late third trimester allows appropriate planning for the management of labour. An ultrasound scan performed at 18–22 weeks of gestation can usually determine the fetal sex and is invaluable in the management of women who are carriers of haemophilia A or B (Figures 7.10 and 7.11). Chorionic villus sampling is the method most commonly employed for prenatal diagnosis of haemophilia. The uptake of prenatal diagnosis and termination of affected pregnancies is low (35% and 50%, respectively), since many carriers of haemophilia, who have family experience of the disorder, do not consider it to be sufficiently disabling to justify termination. In general, in vWD, prenatal diagnosis is offered only to women with severe forms of the disease (for example, type III).

INTRAPARTUM MANAGEMENT

In the absence of any obstetric complication, the optimal mode of delivery for these women is an easy vaginal delivery. Women who will need blood products can usually be identified in the third trimester and an appropriate plan made for their delivery. Following admission in labour or for induction of labour, blood should be sent for a full blood count, including platelet count, coagulation screen and blood grouping. Serum

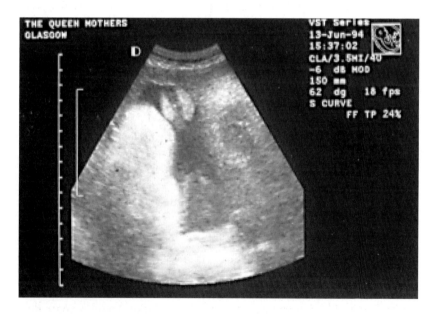

Figure 7.10 Ultrasound scan showing the genitalia of a female fetus; the antenatal determination of fetal sex is important in the management of women who are carriers of haemophilia A or B

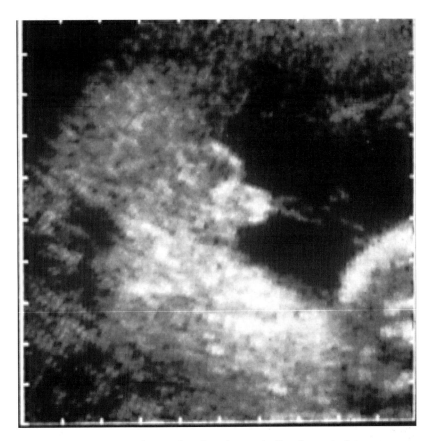

Figure 7.11 Ultrasound scan showing the genitalia of a male fetus

should be retained for cross-matching and appropriate coagulation factors or von Willebrand's factor assays. Carriers of haemophilia who are known to have a male fetus should be delivered by caesarean section if there is a delay in labour and an easy vaginal delivery seems less likely. 'Difficult' forceps deliveries, rotational forceps, ventouse extraction, scalp electrodes or fetal-scalp blood sampling should be avoided if the fetus might have vWD and in haemophilia carriers with a male fetus or where the sex of the fetus is unknown. Caesarean sections or instrumental deliveries should be performed by an experienced obstetrician and every effort should be made to minimise maternal or perineal trauma.

Intravenous or subcutaneous administration of analgesic drugs is preferred in these women and intramuscular injections should be avoided. An epidural can be sited if the coagulation screen is normal, the platelet count greater than $100 \times 10^9/l$ and the Simplate bleeding time less than ten minutes. It has been suggested that these investigations should be repeated before the epidural catheter is removed and, for elective surgery, spinal anaesthesia may be safer.

Maternal bleeding complications with these disorders are usually confined to the intrapartum and postpartum period (including post-termination and post-miscarriage) and there is no evidence of an increased risk of antepartum haemorrhage. The role of blood product therapy in the management of these women has been outlined by a working party of the Haemostasis and Thrombosis Task Force (1994). In summary, the aim is to ensure adequate levels of factor VIII (haemophilia A), factor IX (haemophilia B) or factor VIII and von Willebrand's factor-complex concentrations (vWD) to avoid bleeding complications during delivery and postnatally. Before delivery of the fetus, this will mean infusions of blood products: factor VIII concentrate for haemophilia A, high purity factor IX concentrate for haemophilia B and factor VIII concentrates which contain large amounts of the larger von Willebrand's factor multimers for vWD. Higher levels of clotting factor activity are required for operative deliveries and in the immediate postnatal period (three to four days following vaginal delivery or for four to five days following caesarean section). Carriers of haemophilia A and some patients with type I or type IIA vWD may respond to an infusion of desmopressin by increasing their factor VIII and von Willebrand's factor-complex activities. While there have been concerns regarding the antenatal use of desmopressin, it is now considered satisfactory as it acts on a different receptor subtype from oxytocin and does not appear to stimulate uterine contraction. It may be used after delivery or following miscarriage or termination when a moderate rise in factor VIII activity is required for a short period. Patients with type IIB vWD should not be given desmopressin because of adverse effects on platelets.

POSTPARTUM MANAGEMENT

Neonates should be investigated to determine whether they have inherited the disorder. In view of the physiological changes in the neonate, the diagnosis of some disorders (haemophilia B and vWD) will require repeat investigation at three to six months of age. Intramuscular injections should be avoided in children with vWD and in male children of haemophilia carriers until the diagnosis has been excluded. Vitamin K should be administered orally, immunisation against hepatitis B should be offered and the general practitioner should be informed of the diagnosis and routine immunisations should be given intradermally or subcutaneously. Haematology follow-up should be arranged for the mother and baby.

Thrombocytopenia in pregnancy

In most women the platelet count remains in the normal nonpregnant range during pregnancy. However, mild maternal thrombocytopenia (120–150 × 10⁹/l) is a common finding complicating 5–10% of women at term. The causes of thrombocytopenia in pregnancy are listed in Table 7.27. Guidelines on the management and investigation of thrombocytopenia in pregnancy have been published Letsky and Greaves (1996).

Gestational thrombocytopenia may be associated with a platelet count as low as 50 × 10⁹/l, but it is a benign condition and seems to have no consequences for mother and fetus. A normal platelet count in the early part of pregnancy with a subsequent fall suggests the diagnosis.

INVESTIGATION OF WOMEN WITH THROMBOCYTOPENIA IN PREGNANCY
- Exclusion of drug effects and pre-eclampsia
- Lupus anticoagulant and anticardiolipin antibodies
- Antinuclear factor to exclude connective tissue disease
- Antiplatelet antibodies

Autoimmune thrombocytopenia

Autoimmune thrombocytopenia has an estimated incidence of 1–2 per 10 000 pregnancies and has a female to male ratio of 3 : 1. It is associated with the presence of circulating anti-platelet antibodies, which result in platelet destruction, predominantly in the spleen. Maternal haemorrhage in autoimmune thrombocytopenia is unlikely if the

---

Table 7.27 Causes of thrombocytopenia in pregnancy

- Spurious
- Gestational thrombocytopenia
- Autoimmune idiopathic thrombocytopenia
- Pre-eclampsia and HELLP syndrome
- Disseminated intravascular coagulation
- Haemolytic uraemic syndrome, thrombotic thrombocytopenic purpura
- Folate deficiency
- Other causes, e.g. congenital, systemic lupus erythematosus, infection, drugs

platelet count is greater than $50 \times 10^9/l$ at the time of delivery and haemorrhage unrelated to surgery is unlikely with counts greater than $20 \times 10^9/l$. There is no reliable diagnostic test for autoimmune thrombocytopenia and it remains a diagnosis of exclusion. Laboratory testing for antiplatelet antibodies is not widely available and, when detected, they are not of proven predictive value in pregnancy. Bone marrow examination in autoimmune thrombocytopenia is either normal or megakaryocytic. If there are no suspicious clinical features and the blood count and film reveal thrombocytopenia only, then bone marrow examination is usually unnecessary.

During the antenatal period, if the maternal platelet count is greater than $50 \times 10^9/l$, fortnightly assessment of the platelet count is adequate. Vaginal delivery should be the aim, with delivery by caesarean section for obstetric indications only. Epidural and spinal anaesthesia are best avoided if the platelet count is less than $80 \times 10^9/l$ in view of the risk of haematoma formation. Platelet counts of less than $50 \times 10^9/l$ may be associated with an increased risk of bleeding at the time of delivery and it is recommended that treatment is given to raise the platelet count. Treatment is also indicated if caesarean section is planned to raise the platelet count to more than $80 \times 10^9/l$ to allow regional anaesthesia and also in symptomatic thrombocytopenia when the count is usually less than $20 \times 10^9/l$. The primary treatment options during pregnancy are corticosteroids (60–80 mg of prednisolone daily) and high-dose intravenous human immunoglobulin (IgG). In our own practice we find that IgG infusion is more effective than steroids. They have the additional advantage of blocking antibody transfer to the fetus. Splenectomy, danazol and vinca alkaloids should be avoided during pregnancy. The aim of treatment is to alleviate haemorrhagic symptoms and elevate the platelet count to over $50 \times 10^9/l$. Platelet transfusions should be available during surgery but are recognised to elevate antibody titres. They should not be given until surgery is under way owing to the short lifespan of the transfused platelets.

Although maternal antiplatelet antibodies (IgG) cross the placenta, the risk of severe fetal thrombocytopenia ($<50 \times 10^9/l$) is low ($<10\%$). Antenatal prediction of the fetal platelet count based on the maternal platelet count, antibody titre or splenectomy status, is not accurate, while antenatal cordocentesis or intrapartum fetal scalp sampling is hazardous and should be avoided. Caesarean section has not been shown to improve the fetal outcome. Following delivery, the platelet count is determined from cord blood. If thrombocytopenia is detected, the neonate's clinical and haematological status should be observed closely since the nadir of the platelet count occurs two to five days after delivery, when the splenic circulation becomes established. If the platelet count falls below $20 \times 10^9/l$ or if clinical haemorrhage is apparent, intravenous gammaglobulin is the recommended treatment. Intravenous corticosteroids represent an alternative strategy but are best avoided in the neonate owing to concerns regarding sepsis. Platelet transfusion may be given in the acute situation.

References

Haemostasis and Thrombosis Task Force (1994) Investigation and management of haemorrhagic disorders in pregnancy. *J Clin Pathol* **47**, 100–8

Letsky, E.A. and Greaves, M. (1996) Guidelines on the investigation and management of thrombocytopenia in pregnancy and neonatal alloimmune thrombocytopenia. *Br J Haematol* **95**, 21–6

8 Rhesus disease

Perinatal mortality from haemolytic disease of the newborn (HDN) has been reduced from about 120 per 100 000 live births to 1–2 per 100 000 births in the UK, since the introduction of effective prevention and treatment by anti-D immunoglobulin prophylaxis. The disease does continue to occur and its rarity and consequent lack of experience in its management has led to some potentially avoidable fetal and neonatal morbidity and mortality.

Rhesus blood groups

Approximately 83% of the UK population are rhesus (Rh) D-positive, meaning that they have a protein antigen 'D' on their red blood corpuscles. The remaining 17% who lack this protein are Rh D-negative. When a woman who is Rh D-negative is transfused with Rh D-positive red blood corpuscles she may become immunised by forming an immunoglobulin antibody (IgG) called anti-D, against the D antigen. The anti-D antibody remains permanently in the circulation and destroys any further Rh D-positive red blood corpuscles. Fifteen per cent of women will become sensitised after 1 ml of Rh D-positive red blood corpuscles are administered intravenously and 70–90% after 250 ml. As small a quantity as 0.03 ml of Rh D-positive red blood corpuscles is required to initiate a secondary immune response. The Rh blood group consists of five major antigens (D, C, c, E and e) all of which produce the corresponding clinically important antibodies. The D antigen is 50 times more immunogenic than the other Rh antigens.

Sensitising events during pregnancy

During pregnancy and parturition, small amounts of fetal Rh D-positive red blood corpuscles enter the Rh D-negative mother's circulation. These corpuscles stimulate the production of anti-D IgG1 and IgG3 antibodies, both of which readily cross the placenta and bind to the fetal Rh D-positive red blood corpuscles. Phagocytic cells in the fetal spleen are activated and lyse the fetal red blood corpuscles. Sustained haemolysis results in anaemia, with increased production of red blood corpuscles to compensate. Abnormal production results in erythroblastosis fetalis where primitive red blood corpuscle precursors appear in the circulation. When the anaemia is severe and sustained, the fetus may become hydropic and intrauterine death may ensue. Haemolysis results in excess bilirubin production which, postnatally, leads to jaundice and kernicterus. Maternal exposure to an antigen, during fetomaternal haemorrhage, does not necessarily cause production of an antibody; a series of small immunising doses is more likely to result in the production of antibodies than a large single dose. The most likely time for fetomaternal haemorrhage to occur is at delivery of the fetus and placenta. However, sensitisation can occur following a variety of events during pregnancy and these are listed in Table 8.1 (Figure 8.1). Guidelines for the use of anti-D immunoglobulin have been issued by the Royal College of Obstetricians and Gynaecologists (1999). It is well recognised that a proportion of women develop antibodies during the antenatal period with no recognisable sensitising event.

Prevention of HDN with anti-D immunoglobulin

The protective effect of maternal administration of anti-D immunoglobulin against the development of Rh D sensitisation was demonstrated in the 1960s. This practice has been widely adopted and the incidence of rhesus disease has decreased dramatically. Although there is general agreement on the indications for administration of anti-D immunoglobulin during pregnancy (Table 8.1) there is significant international variation in the dose of anti-D immunoglobulin recommended for routine use. The World Health Organization has

---

Table 8.1 Potential Rh D sensitising events during pregnancy

- Spontaneous miscarriage
- Threatened miscarriage
- Termination of pregnancy
- Ectopic pregnancy
- Amniocentesis
- Chorionic villus sampling
- Antepartum haemorrhage
- External cephalic version

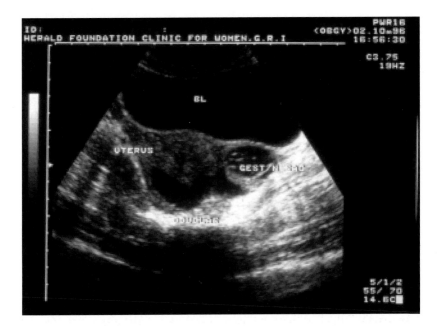

Figure 8.1 Transabdominal ultrasound scan showing an ectopic pregnancy in the left adnexa; anti-D immunoglobulin should be given to all non-sensitised Rh D negative women who have an ectopic pregnancy

recommended that 125 iu of anti-D immunoglobulin should be given per millilitre of fetal red blood corpuscles. It therefore follows that a 500 iu dose is sufficient to cover a fetomaternal haemorrhage of up to 4 ml of red blood corpuscles. In the UK, when a potential sensitising event occurs prior to 20 weeks of gestation, it is current practice to give 250 iu anti-D immunoglobulin and 500 iu after 20 weeks. A Kleihauer test should be performed to identify fetomaternal haemorrhages greater than 4 ml where a larger dose of anti-D immunoglobulin will be required. Anti-D immunoglobulin should be administered within 72–96 hours of the fetomaternal haemorrhage. However, studies have shown that administration up to 13 days post-delivery offers a degree of protection. The introduction of routine immunoprophylaxis with anti-D immunoglobulin has significantly reduced the number of pregnancies complicated by the presence of anti-D antibodies. However, rhesus disease does continue to occur in the UK and new cases of anti-D sensitisation appear to be occurring at a constant rate. The reasons for this are given in Table 8.2.

Table 8.2 Reasons why rhesus disease continues to occur

- Woman already sensitised becoming pregnant
- An inadequate amount of anti-D immunoglobulin given after a sensitising event
- An unrecognised sensitising event
- A clinically occult fetomaternal haemorrhage occurring during pregnancy (common)
- An immunologically Rh D-negative woman ascribed as Rh D-positive
- Immunisation occurring even when an apparently adequate dose of anti-D has been given within the appropriate time (rare)

Red cell immunisation

ANTENATAL SCREENING

It is recommended that all women, regardless of rhesus status, should have their blood tested for red-cell antibodies on two occasions during pregnancy, with the second test being taken in the third trimester. There is a correlation between the gestation at which antibody is first detected and the severity of any resultant HDN. Therefore, if antibodies are detected at booking, they are likely to cause more problems than those detected for the first time later in pregnancy.

In pregnancies where antibodies have been identified, management should include serial monitoring of maternal serum antibody levels throughout pregnancy. It has been recognised for some time that automated quantification of anti-D antibody levels provides more reproducible and meaningful values than manual titration. The level of maternal anti-D immunoglobulin can be used to plan further testing and the need for fetal blood sampling or delivery of the fetus (Table 8.3).

FETAL ASSESSMENT

If the maternal anti-D antibody level is above 10 iu/ml and delivery is not an option because of fetal immaturity, further investigation is necessary. This has included determining the amniotic fluid bilirubin concentration by assessing the amniotic fluid optical density at 453 nm. This technique reflects the degree of fetal haemolysis but not the fetal haemopoietic response and several studies have reported significant discrepancies between the fetal haematocrit and the amniotic fluid optical

Table 8.3 Management based upon maternal anti-D antibody levels; from MacKenzie *et al.* (1991)

Maternal anti-D level (iu/ml)	Repeat maternal anti-D level (weeks)	Fetal blood sampling	Fetal blood transfusion	Likely gestation for delivery (weeks)
<0.5	4	no	no	40
0.5–3.9	2	no	no	40
4.0–9.9	2	no	no	36–38
10–20	2	yes	probably no	33–38
>20	2	yes	probably yes	33–38

density. Analysis of amniotic fluid anti-D concentrations has also been investigated. Although these correlate well with maternal serum anti-D levels, they have no added value in predicting the severity of fetal haemolysis. Fetal assessment by non-invasive methods including fetal movement counting, ultrasound appearances, fetal electrocardiogram waveforms and Doppler ultrasound studies, have not proved helpful in determining whether the fetus will become anaemic. Abnormal fetal heart rate patterns have been described in severe disease. However, cardiotocography (CTG) will identify the seriously anaemic fetus but is not sensitive enough to predict mild to moderate anaemia. Computerised fetal heart rate analysis has identified a consistent relationship between baseline variability and fetal haematocrit and warrants further study.

The only direct method of assessing the severity of rhesus disease is by measuring the haematocrit from fetal blood samples. Several techniques have been described for obtaining antepartum fetal blood, although modern management involves ultrasound guided needling of the umbilical cord, the hepatic vein or the fetal heart. The technique is invasive and associated with late miscarriage or preterm labour in 1–3% in experienced hands. Further, the procedure can result in marked increases in the maternal antibody levels; other reported complications include fetal exsanguination, bradycardia, failure to obtain a sample and cord constriction.

TREATMENT MODALITIES

Intrauterine fetal transfusion was first described in the 1960s by Liley, who performed intraperitoneal transfusion under fluoroscopic screening. This reduced the perinatal mortality rate in severe cases from 95% to 50%. Since then several modifications to the technique have been described, including fetoscopic, then ultrasound, guidance and transfusion directly into the fetal circulation. Intrauterine transfusion is indicated if the fetal haematocrit is less than 25% between 18 and 26 weeks of gestation or less than 30% after 34 weeks of gestation.

The blood used for transfusion should be crossmatched against maternal serum, packed to a haematocrit of 75–90% and screened for hepatitis and cytomegalovirus. The aim of the transfusion is to increase the fetal haematocrit to around 45% and the volume required is calculated from the pretransfusion haematocrit, the donor haematocrit and the estimated fetal blood volume. In some units, premedication is given to the mother for maternal and fetal sedation while others have employed tocolytic agents, antibiotics and corticosteroids. The transfusion may be given directly into the fetal vasculature (umbilical vein, umbilical artery or inferior vena cava), into the fetal heart or into the fetal peritoneal cavity. Transfusions may be required at one- to three-weekly intervals.

COMPLICATIONS OF INTRAUTERINE TRANSFUSION
- Transfusion site trauma
- Haematoma
- Cord spasm
- Umbilical arterial thrombosis
- Fetal thrombocytopenia
- An increase in maternal antibody levels
- Fetal leucoencephalopathy
- Fetal bradycardia

Antenatal prophylaxis for rhesus disease

It is current practice to administer anti-D immunoglobulin to Rh D-negative women following potential sensitising events during pregnancy (Table 8.1). However, it is recognised that 1–2% of all Rh D-negative women show evidence of active Rh D sensitisation despite postnatal prophylaxis, indicating that at least one fetomaternal haemorrhage must have taken place during the antenatal period. One strategy designed to cope with these 'silent' haemorrhages is the routine administration of anti-D immunoglobulin to all Rh D-negative women who have no detectable anti-D antibodies in their blood. A consensus statement in 1998 by the Royal College of Physicians of Edinburgh and representatives of the Royal College of Obstetricians and Gynaecologists reported that routine antenatal anti-D prophylaxis is of proven benefit to significantly reduce levels of Rh D alloimmunisation. At present, however, the dosage and schedule of prophylaxis has not been determined. Two options which both seem effective include a dose of 500 iu at 28 and 34 weeks of gestation or a single larger dose (1500 iu) early in the third trimester. One concern about this strategy is the availability if anti-D immunoglobulin. Anti-D immunoglobulin is a blood product and is concentrated from selected human plasmas containing anti-D antibodies. In the UK, this is collected by plasmapheresis from voluntary, non-remunerated donors who are deliberately sensitised by injection with Rh D-positive red blood corpuscles and their antibody levels repeatedly boosted. The introduction of routine antenatal prophylaxis would more than double the current demand for anti-D immunoglobulin. To fulfil this demand and until a safe monoclonal product is available, existing anti-D donors would have to be maintained at their maximum potential by boosting while more Rh D-negative males and females past childbearing age would have to be recruited for primary immunisation. If there was insufficient anti-D to implement antenatal prophylaxis for all Rh D-negative women, primigravidae should be given priority. The greatest cost benefits of routine anti-D prophylaxis have been demonstrated in primigravid women: a national antenatal prophylaxis programme for primigravidae would cost one-third less than the expected perinatal costs.

Other red cell antibodies in pregnancy

There are many hundreds of red-cell antibodies but few cause severe HDN. The reasons for this include the class of immunoglobulin (only IgG cross the placenta while only IgG1 and IgG3 seem to have a role in HDN) and the immunogenicity of the antigen. The main antibodies of clinical concern are anti-c and anti-Kell, usually from previous transfusion, while about 1/30 ABO-incompatible pregnancies show mild neonatal jaundice.

References

MacKenzie, I.Z., Selinger, M. and Bowell, P.J. (1991) 'Management of red cell isoimmunization in the 1990s' in: J. Studd (Ed.) *Progress in Obstetrics and Gynaecology Volume 9*, pp. 31–53. Edinburgh: Churchill Livingstone

Royal College of Physicians of Edinburgh and Royal College of Obstetricians and Gynaecologists (1998) Joint Consensus Conference on Anti-D Prophylaxis, Proceedings of a joint meeting of the Royal College of Physicians of Edinburgh and Royal College of Obstetricians and Gynaecologists held in Edinburgh, UK, 8–9 April 1997. *Br J Obstet Gynaecol* **105**, Suppl 17

Royal College of Obstetricians and Gynaecologists (1999) *Use of anti-D Immunoglobulin for Rh Prophylaxis*. London: RCOG (Guideline No. 22)

Recommended reading

Chapter 1

Graham, W.J. (1997) Midwife-led care. *Br J Obstet Gynaecol* **104**, 396–8
Hall, M., MacIntyre, S. and Porter, M. (1985) *Antenatal Care Assessed*. Aberdeen: Aberdeen University Press
Hodnett, E.D. (1999) Continuity of caregivers for care during pregnancy and childbirth (Cochrane Review). *The Cochrane Library*, Issue 1. Oxford: Update Software
Royal College of Obstetricians and Gynaecologists (1982) *Report of the RCOG Working Party on Antenatal and Intrapartum Care*. London: RCOG Press
Villar, J. and Khan-Neelofur, D. (1999) Patterns of antenatal care for low-risk pregnancy (Cochrane Review). *The Cochrane Library*, Issue 1. Oxford: Update Software
Wagner, M. (1996) Midwife-managed care. *Lancet* **348**, 208
Walker, P. and James, D.K. (1995) Controversies in management: should obstetricians see women with normal pregnancies? *BMJ* **310**, 36–8

Chapter 2

Barker, D.J.P. and Clark, P.M. (1997) Fetal undernutrition and disease in later life. *Rev Reprod* 2, 105–12
Gardosi, J., Chang, A., Kaylan, B. *et al.* (1992) Customised antenatal growth charts. *Lancet* **339**, 283–7
Greer, I.A. (1999) Thrombosis in pregnancy: maternal and fetal issues. *Lancet* **353**, 1258–65
Gulmezoglu, A.M. and Hofmeyr, G.J. (1999) Maternal nutrient supplementation for suspected impaired fetal growth (Cochrane Review). *The Cochrane Library*, Issue 1. Oxford: Update Software
Holmes, R.P. and Soothill, P.W. (1996) Intrauterine growth retardation. *Curr Opin Obstet Gynecol* **8**, 148–54
Kingdom, J.C.P., Rodeck, C.H. and Kaufmann, P. (1997) Umbilical artery Doppler – more harm than good? *Br J Obstet Gynaecol* **104**, 393–6
Mahadevan, N., Pearce, M. and Steer, P. (1994) The proper measure of intrauterine growth retardation is function, not size. *Br J Obstet Gynaecol* **101**, 1032–5
Manning, F.A., Lange, I.R., Morrison, I. *et al.* (1984) Fetal biophysical profile score and the nonstress test: a comparative trial. *Obstet Gynecol* **64**, 326–31

Neilson, J.P. (1999) Symphysis-fundal height measurement in pregnancy (Cochrane Review). *The Cochrane Library*, Issue 1. Oxford: Update Software

Chapter 3

Burke, G. and Duignan, N.M. (1991) 'Massive obstetric haemorrhage' in: J. Studd (Ed.) *Progress in Obstetrics and Gynaecology Volume 9*, pp. 111–130. Edinburgh: Churchill Livingstone

Fraser, R. and Watson, R. (1989) 'Bleeding during the latter half of pregnancy' in: I. Chalmers, M. Enkin, M.J.N.C. Keirse (Eds) *Effective Care in Pregnancy and Childbirth*. Oxford: Oxford University Press

Love, C.D.B. and Wallace, E.M. (1996) Pregnancies complicated by placenta praevia: what is appropriate management? *Br J Obstet Gynaecol* **103**, 864–7

Macafee, C.H. (1945) Placenta praevia: a study of 174 cases. *J Obstet Gynaecol Br Cwlth* **52**, 313–24

Mouer, J.R. (1994) Placenta praevia: antenatal conservative management, inpatient versus outpatient. *Am J Obstet Gynecol* **170**, 1683–6

Penna, L.K. and Pearce, J.M. (1994) 'Placenta praevia' in: J. Studd (Ed.) *Progress in Obstetrics and Gynaecology Volume 11*, pp. 161–81. Edinburgh: Churchill Livingstone

Chapter 4

Campbell, D.M. (1998) Epidemiology of twinning. *Current Obstetrics and Gynaecology* **8**, 126–34

Dommergues, M., Mahieu-Caputo, D., Mandelbrot, L. *et al.* (1995) Delivery of uncomplicated triplet pregnancies: is the vaginal route safe? A case control study. *Am J Obstet Gynecol* **172**, 513–7

Goldenberg, R.L., Iams, J.D., Miodovnik, M. *et al.* (1996) The preterm prediction study: risk factors in twin gestations. *Am J Obstet Gynecol* **175**, 1047–53

Hanretty, K.P. (1998) Antenatal management of multiple pregnancy. *Current Obstetrics and Gynaecology* **8**, 135–40

Jain, A. and Marlow, N. (1998) Paediatric consequences of multiple pregnancy. *Current Obstetrics and Gynaecology* **8**, 147–52

Landy, H.J., Weiner, S., Corson, S.L. *et al.* (1986) The 'vanishing twin'. Ultrasound assessment of fetal disappearance in the first trimester. *Am J Obstet Gynecol* **155**, 14–19

Murphy, M., Hey, K., Brown, J. *et al.* (1997) Infertility treatment and multiple pregnancy rates in Britain 1938–94. *J Biosoc Sci* **29**, 235–43

Porreco, R., Diss Sabin, E., Heyborne, K.D. *et al.* (1998) Delayed-interval delivery in multifetal pregnancy. *Am J Obstet Gynecol* **178**, 20–3

Sebire, N.J., Snijders, R.J.M., Hughes, K. *et al.* (1997) The hidden mortality of monochorionic twin pregnancies. *Br J Obstet Gynaecol* **104**, 1203–7

Ward, R.H. and Whittle, M. (Eds) (1995) *Multiple Pregnancy*. London: RCOG Press

Webber, L. and Teoh, T.G. (1998) Intrapartum management of multiple gestations. *Current Obstetrics and Gynaecology* **8**, 141–6

Wood, S.L., St Onge, R. and Elliot, P.D. (1996) Evaluation of the twin peak or lambda sign in determining chorionicity in multiple pregnancy. *Obstet Gynecol* **88**, 6–9

Chapter 5

Canadian Preterm Labour Investigators Group (1992) Treatment of preterm labor with the beta-adrenergic agonist ritodrine. *N Engl J Med* **327**, 308–12

El-Sayed, Y.Y., Riley, E.T., Holbrook, H. *et al*. (1999) Randomised comparison of intravenous nitroglycerin and magnesium sulphate for treatment of preterm labour. *Obstet Gynecol* **93**, 79–83

Gibbs, R.S. and Eschenbach, D.A. (1997) Use of antibiotics to prevent preterm birth. *Am J Obstet Gynecol* 177, 375–80

Goldenberg, R.L. and Rouse, D.J. (1998) Prevention of preterm birth. *N Engl J Med* **339**, 313–20

Goodwin, T.M., Paul, R., Silver, H. *et al*. (1994) The effect of the oxytocin antagonist atosiban on preterm uterine activity in the human. *Am J Obstet Gynecol* **170**, 474–8

Higby, K., Xenakis, E.M-J. and Pauerstein, C.J. (1993) Do tocolytic agents stop preterm labor? A critical and comprehensive review of efficacy and safety. *Am J Obstet Gynecol* **168**, 1247–59

Keirse, M.J.N.C. (1995) New perspectives for the effective treatment of preterm labor. *Am J Obstet Gynecol* **173**, 618–28

Lamont, R.F. (1998) New approaches in the management of preterm labour of infective aetiology. *Br J Obstet Gynaecol* **105**, 134–7

Lees, C., Campbell, S., Jauniaux, E. *et al*. (1994) Arrest of preterm labour and prolongation of gestation with glyceryl trinitrate, a nitric oxide donor. *Lancet* **343**, 1325–6

Lockwood, C.J., Seneyi, A.E., Dische, R. *et al*. (1991) Fetal fibronectin in cervical and vaginal secretions as a predictor of preterm labour. *N Engl J Med* **355**, 669–74

Morales, W.J., Smith, S.G., Angel, J.L. *et al*. (1989) Efficacy and safety of indomethacin versus ritodrine in the management of preterm labor, a randomised study. *Obstet Gynecol* **74**, 567–72

Owen, P. and Patel, N. (1995) Prevention of preterm birth. *Baillière's Clin Obstet Gynaecol* **9** (3), 45–79

Papatsonis, D.N.M., van Geizn, H.P., Ader, H.J. *et al*. (1997) Nifedipine and ritodrine in the management of preterm labor, a randomised multicenter trial. *Obstet Gynecol* **90**, 230–4

Scottish Obstetric Guidelines and Audit Project (1997) *The Preparation of the Fetus for Preterm Delivery.* Aberdeen: Scottish Programme for Clinical Effectiveness in Reproductive Health

Taipale, D. and Hiilesmaa, V. (1998) Sonographic measurement of uterine cervix at 18–22 weeks of gestation and the risk of preterm delivery. *Obstet Gynecol* **92**, 902–7

Chapter 6

Broughton-Pipkin, F. (1995) The hypertensive disorders of pregnancy. *BMJ* **311**, 609–13

Chappell, L. and Bewley, S. (1998) Pre-eclamptic toxaemia, the role of uterine artery Doppler. *Br J Obstet Gynaecol* **105**, 379–82

Chappell, L., Seed, P.T., Briley, A.L. *et al.* (1999) Effect of antioxidants on the occurrence of pre-eclampsia in women at increased risk, a randomised trial. *Lancet* **354**, 810–16

CLASP (Collaborative Low-dose Aspirin Study in Pregnancy) Collaborative Group (1994) CLASP, a randomised trial of low dose aspirin for the prevention and treatment of pre-eclampsia among 9364 pregnant women. *Lancet* **343**, 619–29

Davey, D.A. and MacGillivray, I. (1988) The classification and definition of the hypertensive disorders of pregnancy. *Am J Obstet Gynecol* **158**, 892–8

Dekker, G.A. and Sibai, B.M. (1998) Etiology and pathogenesis of pre-eclampsia, current concepts. *Am J Obstet Gynecol* **179**, 1359–75

Douglas, K.A. and Redman, C.W.G. (1994) Eclampsia in the UK. *BMJ* **309**, 1395–1400

Drife, J. and Lewis, G. (Eds) (1998) *Why Mothers Die. Report on Confidential Enquiries into Maternal Deaths in the UK 1994–96.* London: The Stationery Office

Duley, L. (1999) Aspirin for preventing and treating pre-eclampsia, Large trials continue to show no benefit. *BMJ* **318**, 751–2

Eclampsia Trial Collaborative Group (1995) Which anticonvulsant for women with eclampsia? Evidence from the Collaborative Eclampsia Trial. *Lancet* **345**, 1455–63

Greer, I.A. (1996) 'Pregnancy induced hypertension' in: J.S. Cameron, A.M. Davison, J-P. Grunfeld, D.N.S. Kerr and E. Ritz (Eds) *Oxford Textbook of Clinical Nephrology*, 2nd edn. pp. 2349–74. Oxford: Oxford University Press

Greer, I.A. (1999) Thrombosis in pregnancy, maternal and fetal issues. *Lancet* **353**, 1258–65

Pijnenborg, R., Anthony, J., Davey, D.A. *et al.* (1991) Placental bed spiral arteries in the hypertensive disorders of pregnancy. *Br J Obstet Gynaecol* **98**, 649–55

Roberts, J.M. and Redman, C.W. (1993) Pre-eclampsia, more than pregnancy-induced hypertension. *Lancet* **341**, 1447–51

Sattar, N., Bendomir, A., Berry, C. *et al.* (1997) Lipoprotein subfraction concentrations in pre-eclampsia, pathogenic parallels to atherosclerosis. *Obstet Gynecol* **89**, 403–8

Scottish Obstetric Guidelines and Audit Project (1997) *The Management of Mild, Non-proteinuric Hypertension in Pregnancy.* Aberdeen: Scottish Programme for Clinical Effectiveness in Reproductive Health

Sibai, B.M., Ramadan, M.K., Chari, R.S., Friedman, S.A. (1995) Pregnancies complicated by HELLP syndrome, subsequent pregnancy outcome and longterm prognosis. *Am J Obstet Gynecol* **172**, 125–9

Twaddle, S. and Harper, V. (1992) Day care and pregnancy hypertension. *Lancet* **339**, 813–14

Chapter 7

de Swiet, M. (Ed.) (1995) *Medical Disorders in Obstetric Practice*, 3rd edn. Oxford: Blackwell Science

Nelson-Piercy, C. (1997) *Handbook of Obstetric Medicine*. Oxford: Isis Medical Media

(SECTION I)

Garner, P. (1995) Type I diabetes mellitus and pregnancy. *Lancet* **346**, 157–61

Haddow, J.E., Palomaki, G.E., Allan, W.C. *et al*. (1999) Maternal thyroid deficiency during pregnancy and subsequent neuropsychological development of the child. *N Engl J Med* **341**, 549–55

Hall, R., Richards, C.J. and Lazarus, J.H. (1993). The thyroid and pregnancy. *Br J Obstet Gynaecol* **100**, 512–15

Jarrett, R.J. (1993) Gestational diabetes, a non-entity? *BMJ* **306**, 37–8

Mazzaferri, E.L. (1997) Evaluation and management of common thyroid disorders in women. *Am J Obstet Gynecol* **176**, 507–14

O'Doherty, M.J., McElhatton, P.R. and Thomas, S.H.L. (1999) Treating thryotoxicosis in pregnant or potentially pregnant women. The risk to the fetus is very low. *BMJ* **341**, 5–6

Walkinshaw, S.A. (1999) Very tight versus tight control for diabetes in pregnancy (Cochrane Review). *The Cochrane Library*, Issue 1. Oxford: Update Software

(SECTION II)

Sbarouni, E. and Oakley, C.M. (1994) Outcome of pregnancy in women with valve prostheses. *Br Heart J* **71**, 196–201

Thilen, U. and Olsson, S.B. (1998) Pregnancy and heart disease: a review. *Eur J Obstet Gynecol Reprod Biol* **75**, 43–50

(SECTION III)

Holmes, R.C. and Black, M.M. (1982) The specific dermatoses of pregnancy: a reappraisal with special emphasis on a proposed simplified classification. *Clin Exp Dermatol* **7**, 65–73

(SECTION IV)

Brocklehurst, P. (1999) Interventions for reducing mother-to-child transmission of HIV infection (Cochrane Review). *The Cochrane Library*, Issue 1. Oxford, Update Software

Brocklehurst, P. and Rooney, G. (1999) Interventions for treating genital *chlamydia trachomatis* infection in pregnancy (Cochrane Review). *The Cochrane Library*, Issue 1. Oxford, Update Software

European Mode of Delivery Collaboration (1999) Elective caesarean-section versus vaginal delivery in prevention of vertical HIV-1 transmission, a randomised clinical trial. *Lancet* **353**, 1035–9

Gilbert, G.L. (1993) Chickenpox during pregnancy. *BMJ* **306**, 1079–80

Hurtig, A.K, Nicoll, A., Carne, C. *et al.* (1998) Syphilis in pregnant women and their children in the UK: results from national clinician reporting surveys 1994–97.*BMJ* **317**, 1617–19

International Perinatal HIV Group (1999) The mode of delivery and the risk of vertical transmission of human immunodeficiency virus type 1. *N Engl J Med* **340**, 977–87

Johnstone, F.D. (1996) HIV and pregnancy. *Br J Obstet Gynaecol* **103**, 1184–90

Miller, E., Fairley, C.K., Cohen, B.J. *et al.* (1998) Immediate and long term outcome of human parvovirus B19 infection in pregnancy. *Br J Obstet Gynaecol* **105**, 174–8

Silver, H.M. (1998) Listeriosis during pregnancy. *Obstet Gynecol Surv* **53**, 737–40

Welch, J. (1998) Antenatal screening for syphilis: still important in preventing disease. *BMJ* **317**, 1605–6

(SECTION V)

Mahomed, K. (1999) Iron and folate supplementation in pregnancy (Cochrane Review). *The Cochrane Library*, Issue 1. Oxford: Update Software

(SECTION VI)

Girling, J. and de Swiet, M. (1997) Acquired thrombophilia. *Baillière's Clin Obstet Gynaecol* **11** (3), 447–62

Klippel, G.L. and Cerere, F.A. (1989) Rheumatoid arthritis and pregnancy. *Rheum Dis Clin North Am* **15**, 213–39

Le Thi Huong, D., Wechsler, B., Piette, J.C. *et al.* (1994) Pregnancy and its outcome in systemic lupus erythematosus. *Q J Med* **87**, 721–9

Nelson, J.L. and Ostenson, M. (1997) Pregnancy and rheumatoid arthritis. *Rheum Dis Clin North Am* **23**, 195–212

(SECTION VII)

Antonelli, N.M., Dotters, D.J., Katz, V.L. *et al.* (1996) Cancer in pregnancy: a review of the literature. Parts I and II. *Obstet Gynecol Surv* **51**, 125–41

(SECTION VIII)

Moore-Gillon, J. (1994) 'Respiratory disease in pregnancy' in: J. Studd (Ed.) *Progress in Obstetrics and Gynaecology, Volume 11*. pp 111–23. Edinburgh: Churchill Livingstone

Nelson-Piercy, C. and de Swiet, M. (1994) Asthma during pregnancy. *Fetal Mat Med Rev* **6**, 181–9

(SECTION IX)

Davies, M.H., da Silva, R.C.M.A., Jones, S.R. *et al.* (1995) Fetal mortality associated with cholestasis of pregnancy and the potential benefit of therapy with ursodeoxycholic acid. *Gut* **37**, 580–4

Hanan, I.M. (1995) 'Inflammatory bowel disease in pregnancy' in: R.V. Lee, P.R. Garner, W.M. Barron and D.R. Coustan (Eds) *Current Obstetric Medicine, Volume 3*, pp. 43–58. Chicago: Mosby

Nelson-Piercy, C. (1997) Liver disease in pregnancy. *Curr Obstet Gynaecol* **7**, 36–42

(SECTION X)

Johnston, J.W.C., Longmate, J.A. and Frentzen, B. (1992) Excessive maternal weight and pregnancy outcome. *Am J Obstet Gynecol* **167**, 353–72

Watkins, M.L., Scanlon, K.S., Mulinar, E.J. *et al.* (1996) Is maternal obesity a risk factor for anencephaly and spina bifida? *Epidemiology* **7**, 507–12

Wolf, H.M., Zador, I.E., Gross, T.L. *et al.* (1991) The clinical utility of maternal body mass index in pregnancy. *Am J Obstet Gynecol* **164**, 1307–10

(SECTION XI)

Davison, J. (1996) 'Renal complications that may occur in pregnancy' in: J.S. Cameron, A.M. Davison, J-P. Grunfeld, D.N.S. Kerr and E. Ritz (Eds) *Oxford Textbook of Clinical Nephrology*, 2nd edn, pp. 2349–74. Oxford: Oxford University Press

Epstein, F.H. (1996) Pregnancy and renal disease. *N Engl J Med* **335**, 277–8

Jones, D.C. and Hayslett, J.P. (1996) Outcome of pregnancy in women with moderate or severe renal insufficiency. *N Engl J Med* **335**, 226–32

(SECTION XII)

O'Brien, M.D. and Gilmour-White, S. (1993) Epilepsy and pregnancy. *BMJ* **307**, 492–5

Scottish Obstetric Guidelines and Audit Project (1998) *The Management of Pregnancy in Women with Epilepsy*. Aberdeen: Scottish Programme for Clinical Effectiveness in Reproductive Health

(SECTION XIII)

British Society for Haematology (1993) Guidelines on the prevention, investigation, and management of thrombosis associated with pregnancy. *J Clin Pathol* **46**, 489–96

British Thoracic Society (1997) Suspected acute pulmonary embolism: a practical approach. *Thorax* **52** Suppl 4, S1–24

Drife, J. and Lewis, G. (Eds) (1998) *Why Mothers Die. Report on Confidential Enquiries into Maternal Deaths in the United Kingdom 1994–96*. London: The Stationery Office

Economides, D.L., Kadir, R.A. and Lee, C.A. (1999) Inherited bleeding disorders in obstetrics and gynaecology. *Br J Obstet Gynaecol* **106**, 5–13

Greer, I.A. and Walker, I.D. (1996) 'Bleeding in the haemophilia carrier' in: C.D. Forbes, L. Aledort and R. Madhok (Eds) *Haemophilia*, pp. 229–236. London: Chapman and Hall

Greer, I.A. (1997) Epidemiology, risk factors and prophylaxis of venous thrombo-embolism in obstetrics and gynaecology. *Baillière's Clin Obstet Gynaecol* **11**, 403–30

Greer, I.A. (1999) Thrombosis in pregnancy: maternal and fetal issues. *Lancet* **353**, 1258–65

Kadir, R.A., Economides, D.L., Braithwaite, J. *et al.* (1997) The obstetric experience of carriers of haemophilia. *Br J Obstet Gynaecol* **104**, 803–10

Royal College of Obstetricians and Gynaecologists (1995) *Report of the RCOG Working Party on Prophylaxis Against Thromboembolism in Gynaecology and Obstetrics*. London: RCOG Press

Thomson, A.J., Walker, I.D. and Greer, I.A. (1998) Low molecular weight heparin for the immediate management of thromboembolic disease in pregnancy. *Lancet* **352**, 1904

Toglia, M.R. and Weg, J.G. (1996) Venous thromboembolism during pregnancy. *N Engl J Med* **335**, 108–14

Walker, I.D., Walker, J.J., Colvin, B.T. *et al.* (1994) Investigation and management of haemorrhagic disorders of pregnancy. *J Clin Pathol* **47**, 100–8

Wong, V., Cheng, C.H. and Chan, K.C. (1993) Fetal and neonatal outcome of exposure to anticoagulants during pregnancy. *Am J Med Genet* **45**, 17–21

Chapter 8

Duguid, J.K.M. and Bromilow, I. (1994) Value of Kleihauer testing after administration of anti-D immunoglobulin. *BMJ* **309**, 240

Hughes, R.G., Craig, J.I.O., Murphy, W.G. and Greer, I.A. (1994) Causes and clinical consequences of rhesus (D) haemolytic disease of the newborn: a study of a Scottish population, 1985–1990. *Br J Obstet Gynaecol* **101**, 297–300

Liley, A.W. (1961) Liquor amnii analysis in pregnancy complicated by rhesus sensitization. *Am J Obstet Gynecol* **82**, 1359–70

Murphy, K.W. and Whitfield, C.R. (1994) Rhesus disease in this decade. *Contemporary Reviews in Obstetrics and Gynaecology* **6**, 61–7

Robson, S.C., Lee, D. and Urbaniak, S. (1998) Anti-D immunoglobulin in RhD prophylaxis. *Br J Obstet Gynaecol* **105**, 129–34

Index

hypoglycaemia, in diabetic pregnancy 93
hypotension
in pulmonary thromboembolism 159, 160–1
supine 103
hypothyroidism 100–1
hypovolaemia, in placental abruption 34
hypoxia, maternal 106, 131

immune mechanisms, pre-eclampsia 78, 79
immunisation
hepatitis 169, 172
rubella 110–11
immunoglobulin, intravenous human 174, 175
impaired glucose tolerance 95–7
in vitro fertilisation, multiple pregnancy 43–4
indomethacin
adverse effects 66, 67
in polyhydramnios 26
in preterm labour 66
infections 109–18
congenital see congenital infections
in diabetes 91
in obesity 140
preterm labour and 62
in preterm prelabour rupture of fetal membranes 63
urinary tract 109–10, 153
inferior vena cava filters 165
infertility
in epilepsy 146
in prolactinoma 101–2
treatment, multiple pregnancy 43–4, 47–8
inflammatory bowel disease 136–7
INR (international normalised ratio) 165
insulin resistance
in obesity 139, 140
relative, of pregnancy 89
insulin therapy
during labour 95

during pregnancy 90, 93
internal podalic version, in multiple pregnancy 52
intrahepatic cholestasis of pregnancy (ICP) 137–8
intramuscular injections, in inherited bleeding disorders 171, 172
intrapartum management
in asthma 133
in diabetes 94–5
in epilepsy 151
in inherited bleeding disorders 170–2
in multiple pregnancy 49–50
in obesity 142–3
in pre-eclampsia 86–7
in preterm labour 70
intrauterine growth restriction (IUGR) 11–15
adverse outcomes 15
aetiology 13–14
asymmetrical 12
in chronic renal disease 144, 145, 146
definition 12
delivery in 24–5
in diabetes 91
early-onset 18
in heart disease 103
late-onset 18
management 17–18, 19
maternal corticosteroids and 18, 25, 132–3
in pre-eclampsia 82
previous history 15
screening for 15–17
symmetrical 12, 18
in systemic lupus erythematosus 123
see also pre-eclampsia
intrauterine transfusion 181–2
intraventricular haemorrhage 56, 66
iodine
deficiency, relative 98
radioactive 99
iron
deficiency anaemia 119, 120

iron *continued*
  parenteral therapy 120
  serum 120
  supplements 120
isoniazid 134
isoxuprine 65
IUGR *see* intrauterine growth
  restriction

jaundice, neonatal 178, 183

kernicterus 178
Kleihauer test 32, 38, 179
krypton-81m (Kr-81m) 160

labetalol
  for eclampsia 88
  for pre-eclampsia 83–4, 85
labour
  in diabetes 95
  in multiple pregnancy 50, 51–2
  in obesity 142–3
lactate dehydrogenase, serum, in pre-
  eclampsia 80
large for dates pregnancy 25–6
linea nigra 107
lipids, serum, in pre-eclampsia 78
listeriosis 118
liver
  disease 135–8
  pathology, in pre-eclampsia 80
liver function tests 135
  in acute fatty liver of pregnancy
    138
  in intrahepatic cholestasis of
    pregnancy 137
  in pre-eclampsia 80
  in pruritus 107
low molecular weight heparin
  (LMWH)
  adverse effects 164
  in heart disease 105
  in obesity 142, 143
  for thromboprophylaxis 166
  in venous thromboembolism 162–3
low-risk women
  antenatal care providers 2–3

identification 5–8
lung maturity, fetal, in preterm labour
  68–9
lupus, neonatal 126
lupus anticoagulant 124, 125, 127
lupus erythematosus, systemic *see*
  systemic lupus erythematosus

magnesium sulphate
  in myasthenia gravis 154
  for seizure prevention/treatment
    86, 88
magnetic resonance imaging, in
  pulmonary embolism 161, 162
malignancy 128–9
Marfan syndrome 103, 104, 106
maternal deaths, common causes 81
maternal serum screening
  in diabetic pregnancy 94
  in multiple pregnancy 48
mean cell haemoglobin (MCH) 119,
    120
mean corpuscular haemoglobin
  concentration (MCHC) 119
mean corpuscular volume (MCV) 119
meconium staining, in intrahepatic
  cholestasis of pregnancy 137
metabolic rate, maternal 129
methimazole 99
methyldopa, for pre-eclampsia 83, 84,
    85, 87
midwives 2–3
miscarriage
  in chronic renal disease 145
  in multiple pregnancy 45
  in obesity 139
  recurrent 127
  in systemic lupus erythematosus
    122
mitral stenosis 104, 105
mobility, restricted, in obesity 142
monoamniotic placentation 44–5
monochorionic twinning 44, 45, 46–7
multigravidae, risk scoring 7
multiple pregnancy 43–53
  complications 45–7
  epidemiology 43–4